From TB to AIDS

SUNY Series in Afro-American Studies

John Howard and Robert C. Smith, Editors

From TB to AIDS

Epidemics among Urban Blacks since 1900

David McBride

State University of New York Press

A AY 8076

Published by
State University of New York Press, Albany

© 1991 State University of New York

For information, address State University of New York
Press, State University Plaza, Albany, N.Y., 12246

Production by M. R. Mulholland
Marketing by Bernadette LaManna

Library of Congress Cataloging in Publication Data

McBride, David, 1949–
      From TB to AIDS : epidemics among urban Blacks since 1900 / by
David McBride.
            p. cm. — (SUNY series in Afro-American studies)
      Includes bibliographical references.
      Includes index.
      ISBN 0-7914-0528-1 (alk. paper). — ISBN 0-7914-0529-X (pbk. :
alk. paper)
      1. Afro-Americans—Diseases. 2. Afro-American—Health and
hygiene. 3. Social medicine—United States. 4. Epidemiology.
I. Title. II. Series.
      [DNLM: 1. Blacks—history—United States. 2. Communicable
Diseases—history—United States. 3. Delivery of Health Care-
-history—United States. 4. Disease Outbreaks—history—United
States. 5. Prejudice—United States. 6. Urban Population—history-
-United States. WA 11 AA1 M35f]
RA448.5.N4M39   1991
616' .0089'96073—dc20
DNLM/DLC
for Library of Congress   90–9758
                                                                                 CIP

10 9 8 7 6 5 4 3 2 1

Contents

Illustrations

Tables

Figures

Preface

In this book I describe the nature and sociomedical perceptions of the diseases that most gravely affected America's black population from the beginning of this century to the late 1980s. The first part of the study looks at the ways that the nation's medical, public health, and African-American communities came to grips with mass disease outbreaks that appeared to strike black populations especially hard. As the New Deal and World War II decades unfolded, the federal government took the lead in addressing the higher mortality levels that African-Americans experience. This ascendency of federal government health agencies came at the same time America's inner-city black communities became storehouses of physical and political despair, often outside the reach of federal health care initiatives. In the second part of this study I trace how national government approached the health problems of black communities. But I also show how key medical and social welfare authorities, as well as lay groups, diverged markedly in dealing with the health problems of blacks, depending on whether their vantage point was rooted in black community health professions and activism.

Few medical historians accept the assumption that medical progress and setbacks in controlling disease are to be measured solely by a narrow stream of clinical data amassed on individual patients, and the deeper understanding of biological disease processes and therapies that usually ensues. In this book, I have used a multiangled approach that may at first blush test the flexibility of the strict specialist or generalist. My goal was to measure the effects of disease outbreaks and race–health differentials on black Americans as well as expert structures *within* and *outside* of black communities involved in controlling this problem. Hence, I was compelled to look not only into the thinking, actions, and programs that emerged from mainstream medical, social science, and government health institutions, but also less-visible black medical, social work, and lay sectors as well.

I owe special thanks to the Rockefeller Foundation, which provided a postdoctoral research grant that allowed me time away from my teaching and other university duties to travel widely throughout the nation's libraries, archives, and medical institutions. While I owe gratitude to all of the institutions I visited for archival and library materials (each is identified in the notes), I must single out the staffs of the Moorland-Spingarn Research Center at Howard University, the Amistad Research Center at Tulane University in New Orleans, the State University of New York Health Science Center Library at Syracuse, and the Francis A. Countway Library of Medicine in Boston, Massachusetts. Much of the research for this book was completed while I was a visiting scholar at the National Library of Medicine in Bethesda, Maryland. To John Parascandola and his staff at the NLM's Division of History, many thanks. Monroe H. Little, Cyril Griffith, Edna B. McKenzie, Aida Louise Harris, and Charles L. Blockson took time from their busy schedules whenever I approached them for general advice or research tips regarding my project. Peggy Gifford and Megeen Mulholland, editors at the State University of New York Press, were patient and responsive throughout all the stages of this work. My colleagues and students at the State University of New York–Binghamton where I have been fortunate to teach during most of the 1980s also inspired me throughout this project. Finally, the deepest root of this book lies in the encouragement and support I have received over the years from my family. Throughout the years of this project Patrice and Julian, my two small sons, carried on an aggressive yet enjoyable debate with me about their strong preferences for baseball and snowball fights. Ruth McBride Jordan, my mother, was her usual helpful self. Others who assisted me with dispatch included Dennis, Rosetta, Billy, Rose, Helen, Gary, Ricardo, Debbie, James Charles, Dorothy, Kathy, Judy, Hunter, and Henry. Views of fact and interpretation throughout this book are, of course, mine alone.

Introduction

Opening the Historical Path

1

Throughout the 1980s, the acquired immune deficiency syndrome (AIDS) epidemic caused tremendous destruction to many segments of American society. Currently it appears that low-income blacks and Hispanics are experiencing the highest proportional mortality from this disease. Although blacks and Hispanics comprised only a small percentage of America's population, by 1988 seventy-eight percent of the pediatric cases of AIDS were black or Hispanic, as were 71 percent of the female cases.[1] Moreover, United States Surgeon General C. Everett Koop suggested in a 1988 interview that a fundamental problem in communication existed between the medical experts and the black community. According to Koop, the new wave of minority victims had been "difficult to address largely because of the [poverty] situation, [and] also because it is difficult in our society, even in people who are in public health who are aware of it, to get a message that hits that population."[2]

Analysis of the historical dimension underlying the AIDS crisis in African-American society and culture has not yet emerged from the wide range of social scientific and medical literature that has appeared. Indeed, the health history of post-Emancipation African-Americans generally has had a minor place in recent American medical history, historical sociology and medical anthropology. What little current historiography there is on late nineteenth- and twentieth-century black Americans focuses primarily on the integration of the medical professions and health care facilities. The consensus within this scholarship is that slavery and racial segregation in early American socioeconomic and political development planted a deeply rooted racial divide in American medical life. The segregation of hospitals, medical education and professions, and unequal allocation of health care facilities are all chiefly the by-product of the general civil

and economic discrimination that black Americans faced following
the demise of Reconstruction. Segregation in the health care sphere,
as in other major public institutions, waned during the middle of the
twentieth century. It was during this period that the civil rights
movement began to affect America's health system, resulting in substantial racial integration in hospital admission policies and staffing.
Also during this era liberalized health financing and a greater number of blacks achieving middle-class status, resulted in blacks gaining greater access to medical care services.

When looking back at the health history of black America,
however, we see one pattern that has yet to be addressed squarely
in recent African-American or medical historical scholarship: the persistently higher mortality and morbidity levels for black Americans in
many major disease categories when the levels for the general American population have been declining significantly. This excess black
mortality and morbidity, furthermore, has appeared even throughout
periods when medical care technology or political integration, or
both, have been advancing. For instance, from 1900 to the 1920s,
when specialized medicine and public hygiene movements were
accelerating throughout the nation, the tuberculosis (TB) epidemic
among urban blacks emerged as the most urgent public health concern among municipal health authorities, social welfare workers, and
the medical community (practitioners and researchers). In these
decades, when the black population of the major cities spiraled
upward, annual mortality among blacks, usually from TB, was two
to four times higher than those of whites. Other infectious diseases
also took a much higher toll on blacks. Black urban and rural death
rates from syphilis, malaria, influenza, and puerperal causes, for
example, ran generally two or three times higher for blacks than
whites.[3]

Through the Depression and World War II decades a similar
black–white health differential prevailed, despite the overall decline
in infectious disease-related mortality, the rise of potent chemotherapies and broadened use of seroepidemiology, and the emergence of
federal health care initiatives that substantially increased health services for the nation's working-class and poor sectors. Black mortality
and morbidity rates from venereal disease, as well as those related
to malnutrition greatly outdistanced those of whites. From 1929 to
1931, for example, the black death rate from pellegra exceeded
whites' ten to one, and was six to one in 1939–41.[4] By the 1960s,
when so-called degenerative diseases, such as coronary heart diseases and cancer, had eclipsed infectious diseases as the nation's

leading killers, blacks again were experiencing significantly higher infectious disease-related death rates.[5] Once again, this health–race discrepancy prevailed during a time when both the integration and availability of medical care services expanded.

Currently, much of the nation's black community remains threatened by serious, largely preventable health and social ills. Among the most severe medical and related social problems facing blacks are disproportionately high levels of (1) infant and maternal mortality; (2) teenage pregnancy; (3) behavioral disorders; (4) mortality and community disorder linked to violent crime and drug abuse; (5) cancer and cardiovascular disease; and (6) most recently, AIDS.[6]

Historians and other social scientists of American health have provided a general description of the strong role that racial discrimination played in determining black Americans' access to medical care during the first two-thirds of this century. Moreover, two fine studies have recently appeared that examine the medical education and health problems of southern blacks.[7] Researchers have yet to produce, however, historical sociologies of the broad health patterns unfolding in urban African-American society, or of the medical and public perceptions of these black city-dwellers' health problems. Nor have they described the ways in which these perceptions shaped health care and social welfare policy aimed at reducing the high mortality rates of black Americans from disease. Indeed, except for the integration question, current scholarship is so sparse on sociomedical developments and health patterns of urban blacks that it provides virtually no background upon which to assess the current diffusion of AIDS throughout the black community, or the critical gap that exists between AIDS prevention and treatment programs, on the one hand, and black populations who need these services, on the other.[8]

The lack of historical studies regarding the role of disease and alienation in shaping the twentieth century urban black experience is especially glaring when one considers the exciting strides biological and social historians, demographers, and medical anthropologists recently have made charting the impact of epidemics, disease, nutrition and environment on premodern peoples and New World slave societies.[9] In contrast to these advances, the modern development of African-Americans has been explained by historians almost exclusively within three conceptual frameworks: segregation versus integration of blacks throughout formal political and educational institutions; class versus race factors as the primary shapers of black

Americans' status; and, to a lesser and relatively unexplored extent, gender factors molding the experiences of black women.[10]

But what about the origins and ever-present social impact of disease and sickness, and the concomitant technological upbuilding of the modern health care establishment, on post-Reconstruction, urban black America—phenomena that do not fit neatly into any of these three frameworks? Do not the current extraordinarily high level of AIDS, widespread drug abuse, and similar health problems throughout many black communities underscore this question? On these issues, the social history and policy studies literature is virtually silent.

My study attempts to address this gap in the literature. It challenges particularly the overuse of the "segregation to integration" and "class-over-race" typologies to interpret contemporary black American medical history. While useful for explaining black admissions to medical professions and facilities, and the impact of economic stratification within modern black American society, they are but a pair of one-dimensional perspectives that fail to reach into the private worlds of black social (physical) existence. Both perspectives have shortcircuited historical investigation of three interrelated social foundations: the physical, the cultural and the medical. Hence, we have little understanding of the health dimension of the twentieth-century black American experience—the precedents for the AIDS crisis, and the black–white health differential, for instance—and the ways that the medical, public health, and state sectors absorbed and refracted these health patterns. I shall demonstrate that in the coming decades, alongside race, class, and gender, the role of disease will have to be illuminated if we are to acknowledge fully the social history of modern black America.

2

In historicizing disease and emergent contemporary African-American society, I pursue three "signpost" questions: (1) What was the nature and extent of epidemic disease and other mass illness among black Americans throughout the course of this century? (2) Why did medical and sociopolitical segments in both the white and black communities interpret and address these health problems of blacks the way they did? (3) What did this sociomedical response, in the form of intellectual constructions and social welfare and policy movements, mean to the larger social and cultural development of modern African-American and American society?

Answers to these questions entail neither merely recounting discrete "big" events, nor depicting a simple, linear health progress. Indeed, the argument advanced here is that these signposts stemmed from four simultaneous and fluid "revolutions." The first revolution was the physical-environmental transplanting of African-Americans from primarily rural and small-urban regions of the South, to industrial economies and household environments in the nation's largest metropolises. Second, there was a radical shift for blacks in relationship to the rise of the modern health care establishment: they changed from an underserved peripheral body to a central client population within American medicine and public health, as the health care system evolved from clusters of unevenly defined professions and institutions, to one of the the country's most socially and economically powerful human service industries. Third, epistemological cycles emerged that broadened the appeal of an error-ridden medicotheoretical orientation (or paradigm) that linked disease causally to "race" or black African descent. Finally, most white and black Americans' cultural experiences diverged as the traditional (pre-twentieth-century) lines of sociopolitical segregation were reshaped to run intricately throughout the urban-industrial context.

To answer the three signpost questions, I advance a twofold thesis. First, as the twentieth century progressed, the black health experience moved to the center of fundamentally conflicting epidemiological orientations, that is, competing "epidemic paradigms," that had been laid down during the first half of this century.[11] Second, following World War II the black medical and social welfare communities, to address the health crises of inner-city and poor rural black communities, attempted to unify their epidemic paradigms with those of the larger medical and health politics community.

The upcoming chapters show that this tridimensional split in the sociomedical response to sickness confronting blacks—among the mainstream medical establishment, black and white medical caregivers serving largely black clientele, and the social movements and indigenous health culture and practices of black working-class communities—had been formed over decades. It is this separation that is currently hampering the overall mission of American health care to eliminate the AIDS crisis of urban black Americans. This conflict between medical paradigms and the black health and social problems of yesterday will have to be identified and harmonized before the nation can curtail the AIDS epidemic currently gripping black American communities. This study follows the historical path to the origins of this conflict.

3

To begin investigation into black contemporary health history from the beginning of the twentieth century to the current AIDS crisis, I shall focus on epidemics. Contemporary medicine and social science have conventionally defined epidemics as sharp jumps in mortality and morbidity caused by so-called infectious or communicable diseases.[12] More recently, epidemic has come to denote also rapid expansion in degenerative disease rates, unhealthy social behavioral trends, or alienation involving extraordinary waves of violence, juvenile delinquency, and self-abuse.[13] I focus primarily on the conventional type, that is, communicable disease outbreaks, for two reasons. First, the social and medical responses to the major infectious diseases early in this century developed into competing paradigms. These medical and public health "explanatory models" dominated the disease-control policies instituted during later epidemics in post–World War II urban black America.[14] Second, it was these earlier orientations that established limits on the black community's medical and social leadership as they attempted to mobilize the nation against communicable-disease epidemics and other mass illness among inner-city black communities.

Before the AIDS crisis there were three critical waves of disease that struck the black American population. Chapters 1, 2, and 3 will cover the period from the beginning of the century through the 1920s when TB was the infectious disease taking the heaviest toll on blacks. Chapter 4 will focus on the Depression and New Deal eras when venereal disease moved to the top of the nation's concerns for black health, and when the huge federal health care machine emerged. Chapter 5 will cover the 1940s through the 1970s when mobilization for World War II and sprawling urbanization inspired broader federally supported "wars" on communicable diseases, especially on TB and venereal disease. Finally, Chapter 6 will concentrate on the 1980s when the black poor throughout the nation experienced the third wave of severe health problems and care gaps that increasingly powered and was powered by the AIDS epidemic.

Part I

Discovering the Black Health Crisis

Chapter 1

The Southern Negro Problem
and the Origins of Sociomedical Racialism

Historians of the African-American experience and American race relations characterize the turn of the century as a sociopolitical and economic low point for the black citizenry. It is a time when there is a "triumph of white supremacy" in the post-Reconstruction South (according to the works of John Hope Franklin), a sociopolitical and legal "nadir" for blacks (Rayford Logan), "retrogressionist" cultural beliefs about blacks (Herbert Gutman) and an ascendency of "conservative" segregationism (Joel Williamson).[1] But these are only the broad strokes, an outline of constraints on black American life through the Gilded Age. The finer features within this big picture reveal expanding, sometimes frantic, miniature developments within government, education, social welfare agencies and police institutions to govern the spiraling, turn-of-the-century African-American mass.*

As black, native white and new European immigrant Americans underwent the initial jolts of modern urbanization, the Progressive Era expert sector took shape. This rising network of medical, public health, and social welfare professionals came to recognize that a severe black–white health discrepancy existed. Contagious diseases

---

*To call attention to subtle shifts in scientific, popular, and regional terms for African-Americans or blacks, I have retained the exact spelling of the word Negro (which was sometimes spelled with a lowercase "n") as it appeared in the original source. Sterling Stuckey, a leading authority on American culture and race relations, emphasizes that at the end of the nineteenth century, African-Americans preferred to capitalize Negro, while regarding "the lowercase spelling as an insult to their people." See his chapter, "Identity and Ideology: The Names Controversey," in his seminal work, *Slave Culture: Nationalist Theory and the Foundations of Black America* (New York: Oxford University Press, 1987), 193–244.

such as diphtheria, typhus, tuberculosis (also called TB or consumption) and, to a lesser extent, syphilis, emerged as the most serious
threats to public health in the United States. The technical dominion
and professional authority of the Progressive Era municipal and
social welfare sector rested on gaining the public's trust that it could
ameliorate such health problems and the social ills of industrializa-
tion and urban growth. With blacks increasingly populating urban
America and their disease rates presumably high, by World War I
many public health and social service experts in medicine, education, industry, and government believed that the future of America
depended on proper understanding and resolution of the black
health "threat."

Throughout the Progressive Era, then, municipal and social
work leaders aggressively investigated and collected data on the
physique, health, psychological characteristics, and crime patterns of
black Americans. In medicine, the black health problem compound-
ed existing professional insecurity and scientific woes. Establishing
more effective etiologies and therapeutic approaches to TB and
syphilis in general was seriously frustrating early twentieth century
clinical and public health investigators. Now the ubiquitous blacks
seemed to be especially subject to the destructiveness of these diseases. Most white medical authorities believed that high black
American mortality rates from TB and syphilis, were caused by racial
characteristics that could be explained by traditional syphilology,
pathology, and social Darwinism. In the meantime, from within the
lay black community and black medical profession, a largely voluntary public health movement emerged to curtail the spread of TB
and other contagious health threats.

1

From the turn of the century to the mid-1910s, vital statistics
and epidemiological data on the health of blacks were sparse. But by
the end of World War I a crescendo of statistics grew supporting the
idea that blacks posed a major public health menace.[2] Five types of
piecemeal data provided a generally grim picture of the death rates
and health problems of black Americans: census returns on mortality
of limited geographic areas; data provided by the United States Army
on rejected applicants and enlistees; census reports on insane, blind,
and deaf populations (then considered "sick and defective" groups);
vital statistics provided by certain municipalities, counties or states;
and morbidity reports of large hospitals.[3] Overall mortality for blacks

in 1900 stood at 29.6 deaths per 1,000 population compared to 17.3 for whites.[4] According to the report of the annual Conference for the Study of the Negro Problems held at Atlanta University in 1906, the topic of which was the health status of blacks, this mortality data also showed the "greatest enemy of the black race is consumption."[5] The TB death rate for blacks in 1900 was nearly triple that of whites (485 to 174 deaths per 100,000 respectively). The next four most frequent killers of blacks were pneumonia (356 compared to 185 for whites), diseases of the nervous system (308 to 214), typhoid fever (68 to 32), and malaria (63 to 7).[6]

Of these five leading causes for black mortality, one, the vaguely defined "nervous disorders," is degenerative (or noninfectious) and typically the end-effects of heart problems like atherosclerosis or cerebrovascular disease (stroke). Three others, typhoid fever, malaria, and pneumonia are infectious. These latter three illnesses have distinct, dramatic symptoms that appear in a matter of days. They are strongly associated with immediate environmental conditions. Typhoid fever is linked to unsanitary food products (especially milk) or water supplies, while malaria is vector-borne (transmitted by insects).[7] Influenza-pneumonia in its acute phase normally lasts from three to five days and frequently occurs as a local outbreak in a close-knit setting of people such as households, prisons, army training camps, or orphanages.[8]

As the twentieth century opened, TB posed the most persistent danger to the nation's black communities. TB stood above the four other leading causes of deaths in its uniquely complex symptomology and the severe socioeconomic damage it rendered. The disease created social havoc because it tended to strike individuals in the most productive phase of their life. Robert Koch (1843–1910), a precursor of bacteriology and discoverer of the tubercle bacillus, wrote that "[i]f the number of victims which a disease claims is the measure of its signficance, then all diseases, particularly the most dreaded infectious diseases, such as bubonic plague, Asiatic cholera, etc., must rank far behind tuberculosis." Koch estimated that about one-seventh of all humans died from TB, and, if "one considers only the productive middle-age groups, tuberculosis carries away one-third and often more of these."[9] Following infection, the risk of developing clinical TB varies highly. Also, the interval between the period of initial infection and the emergence of definite symptoms and debilitation may span a few weeks to decades. Today TB still ranks near the top among the world's leading causes of disability and mortality.[10]

Just as these early mortality reports brought into focus the serious threat TB posed to blacks, the results of physical examinations on rejected military applicants and army personnel signaled a warning that venereal disease among blacks was comparatively high. The ratio of blacks and whites rejected by the military from 1901 to 1904 for key disorders revealed that blacks had annual venereal disease rates roughly 50 to 250 percent higher than those of whites. Atlanta University researchers, however, were careful to point out that military morbidity data for enlistees revealed that in some cases whites evidenced higher venereal diseases rates than blacks.

Data of 1904 on roughly 60,000 white and black troops, for example, contained a significant number of soldiers who had served in foreign countries such as the Philippines, Cuba, or Puerto Rico. These military records disclosed that the prevalence of venereal disease was about 25 percent higher for whites (109) than blacks (87). According to the Atlanta University proceedings, this discrepancy not only indicated obvious miscegenation, but also exposed the hypocrisy of linking venereal disease to alleged race traits of Negroes such as biological susceptibility or moral promiscuity. "[I]n venereal disease the foreign service of white troops has led to their excess," the proceedings state, "a curious commentary on imperialism."[11]

Mortality statistics available for some major cities for the years 1884 to 1900 also suggested that during the opening decade of this century, black mortality was substantially higher than that of whites.[12] Consumption death rates in 1900 for blacks in Boston, Washington, D.C., Baltimore, and New York were 742 (per 100,000), 514, 448, and 503, respectively. By contrast the overall TB mortality rate for whites (in registration areas) in 1900 was 174.[13]

Gradually during the 1900s and 1910s municipalities, counties, and states passed vital statistics laws which established units within their health boards or general administrations for the specific function of collecting birth, stillbirth, and death statistics on a regular basis. The quality and extent of such units varied greatly from locale to locale, as the personnel and methods for their collection, mortality classification for these statistics, and ultimate benefit of this data were still defined differently by each locale or state.[14] Some jurisdictions collected data weekly, others monthly, all did so annually. As this data grew, public health authorities and medical societies became more aware of the black–white mortality differential and were usually the first to interpret this data for their political and lay communities.[15]

These local vital statistics also showed TB death rates for blacks to be extraordinarily high. Typical was the report for June

1911 by the Board of Health of New Orleans. It indicated that of the 258 deaths of blacks in the city that month, TB was the leading killer (45), followed by heart disease (34), diarrhea, dysentery and enteritis (28), and Bright's disease (kidney disorder, 25). As for New Orleans's whites, there had been 375 deaths, with heart disease the leading cause of death (55) followed by diarrhea (52), Bright's disease (40), and TB (35).[16] In Birmingham, Alabama, mortality information gathered annually by its registrar of vital and mortuary statistics, combined with information from other sources (such as private anti-TB organizations), disclosed a shocking discrepancy in TB mortality along racial lines. From 1905 to 1915 the average TB death rate was 80 (per 100,000) for white residents of Birmingham compared to 390 for blacks.[17]

When statewide vital statistic offices were created, they provided another stream of information pointing to an extremely high death toll for blacks from TB. Indeed, the need for organized data on black health for counties and states with large concentrations of blacks was a prime rationale for initiating offices to pursue what was then called the "science of vital statistics."[18] Among the first states to set up a vital statistics office in the South was Virginia, which passed its law in 1912 and collected its first statewide vital statistics in 1913.[19] Although Virginia had been admitted to the federal census registration area in 1913, state health authorities still believed that a substantial number of births and deaths were still being overlooked. They stated that their new vital statistics unit was especially significant because its annual report would be "the first published by any American State [sic] in which there is so large a negro element—so serious a factor in public health—as large as in Virginia."[20]

Health officials of Virginia were not surprised to find that TB death rates among black residents exceeded greatly those of whites. The 1913 data for nine of Virginia's largest cities which included Richmond (populated by 84,401 whites and 48,784 blacks), Norfolk (53,374 and 29,825), and Portsmouth (23,708 and 12,788), indicated blacks were dying from TB at over three times the rate of whites.[21] "At the outset, then," according to Virginia's vital statistics report for that year, "we find in the city negro the direst sufferer from tuberculosis [while the] white citizen of these urban communities suffers lightly by comparison."[22]

The tone of fatalism that Virginia health authorities cast on the health plight of black Virginians was especially evident in a section of the 1913 report, "Deaths in the Commonwealth." It disclosed a mortality rate for blacks substantially higher than its birth rate. Statewide the black birth-to-death rate differential was 5.7 per thousand annually (23.9 to 18.2), but for whites 14.8 (26.6 to 11.8). In the urban areas, the health authorities found, "the colored race is losing more rapidly than it is gaining."[23] The urban black death rate exceeded the birth rate, 26.8 to 19.9; while these rates for urban whites were essentially the reverse, a death rate of 14.8 to a birth rate of 21.9. Such figures, if assumed accurate, according to Virginia health authorities "presage the extinction of the negro in the cities of Virginia."[24]

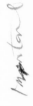

Although state and federal reports on vital statistics contained bits of information that indicated especially healthy aspects of black populations, the medical and public health establishment tended to overemphasize the high black death rates.[25] John W. Trask, assistant surgeon general of the United States Public Health Service, called attention to this tendency in a paper delivered at the American Public Health Convention in Rochester, New York, during 1915. Discussing the interpretation of mortality rates of the black populations, Trask urged that public health researchers explore more specific reasons for the high black death rate and "whether the factors which produce the difference in the death-rates can be removed and the colored death-rate lowered until it approximates that of the white element of the population."[26]

Trask further recommended that black mortality rates of southern states and large cities be compared to those of smaller populations, rural populations, and to death rates of European (white) foreign countries. Finally, he argued that economic or industrial differences of a particular region's black and white populations evidencing wide mortality gaps be explored to measure the ill effects of these factors. His own preliminary survey of federal census mortality data demonstrated that rural white and black populations frequently had only small mortality differentials, that age-distribution affected mortality strongly, and that the black mortality rate (in 1912) essentially equaled those of "the white populations of Hungary, Roumania, Spain, and Austria."[27] In light of these findings, he advised against a bedrock faith in the conclusion that "there was in the colored race some peculiar characteristic which caused it to have a death-rate higher than that for a white population similarly located."[28]

Trask's voice, however, like those of the Atlanta University study group's a few years earlier, represented only a minor opinion compared to the dominant medical thought which linked race to the high infectious disease rates of black Americans. Dr. J. S. Fulton, a secretary of the Maryland Board of Health, rejected the intent of Trask's paper, stating that it "would require a more critical study" of the mortality data. While the points Trask made to deemphasize the race factor were interesting and "advantageous to the negro to believe," Fulton commented bluntly, "the assumption of defective racial adaptation is . . . not easily disposed of."[29]

The way in which the nation's medical, public health, and charitable sectors conceptualized and responded institutionally to the high prevalence of TB and syphilis among black Americans, provided the rough foundation for approaches to black health problems of later decades. This early idea system or epidemic imperative, combining biological and sociological notions that blacks were biologically most susceptible to primary infectious diseases, reflects that mainstream American society through the World War I decade generally viewed black Americans more as a source of contagion than as fellow victims.

2

Not only were TB and syphilis among the leading killers of the day; they also posed etiological and epidemiological terrains that were virtually impregnable. TB is usually spread by inhalation of airborne droplets secreted by persons usually severely diseased and who have tubercle bacilli in their sputum. Causal pathogens for TB had been identified by the historic bacterial laboratory research of Koch and his generation. Yet neither this basic research nor the larger community of clinicians could unravel ways to cut the spread of these diseases by human carriers.[30] Several decades of international research and prevention campaigns had to pass before TB and syphilis could be managed effectively. Moreover, it would take many decades for populations in America to build up natural immunities to TB and other infectious diseases.

In the meantime, as World War I approached, social Darwinism, eugenics, and Euronationalism stormed across the Atlantic into the American intellectual terrain.[31] The initial stream of vital statistics and military medical records on black mortality and morbidity blended into an explosion of medical, psychological, and demographic studies on the negative effects of darker races and black Americans on larger society.[32] These academic studies and popular scientific diatribes centered on establishing a fundamental connection between phenotypical race traits and mental illness, criminality, and low intelligence, as well as black (and, to a limited extent, foreign-born and female) biological inferiority and susceptibility to infectious disease.[33]

At the turn of the century, no demographic or sociological researcher enunciated the racialist idea that black Americans were an inferior, even "dying," race so authoritatively as the health statistician, Frederick L. Hoffman. His 1896 study *Race Traits and Tendencies of the American Negro,* and the clinical work *The Surgical Peculiarites of the Negro* by the eminent southern surgeon Rudolph Matas, became standard references for medical and sociological research through World War I postulating race distinctions as the basis for the black–white health discrepancy.[34]

Hoffman, whom Herbert Gutman describes as an "influential racial Darwinist," brought together the central threads of the "dying race" concept.[35] These diachronic racialist concepts postulated that (1) slavery had had a civilizing effect on black Africans: "All the facts brought together . . . prove that the colored population is gradually parting with the virtues . . . developed under the regime of slavery"; (2) blacks possessed a "race or constitutional trait" for psychological disintegration and an "immense amount of immorality" from which syphilis and tuberculosis "are the inevitable consequences"; and (3) even if these factors did not exist, evolution in the tropical climate and uncivilized conditions made the gradual "extinction of the [Negro] race" inevitable.[36]

During the opening decades of the twentieth century, Hoffman exercised great influence in the area of population studies of cancer. To his credit, he was one of the first influential statisticians to discount the theory that cancer was primarily an hereditary or infectious disease.[37] Instead, he stressed environmental and geographical factors (such as "a civilized mode of life") that encouraged contact with irritants causing the disease, as well as distance of populations from the equator. "Native races" living near the equator ate simpler foods and wore looser clothes. "The almost non-occurrence of breast cancer among the women of primitive races" was because "[p]ractically all the women of native races live simple lives, are undernourished rather than overnourished, and wear clothing consisting of a single [loose] garment."[38]

But Hoffman also framed his environmental cancer theories within a racialist conception, urging that the white race was more prone to cancer than the Negro one. In 1913 he told members of the American Gynecological Society meeting in Washington, D.C., that "[t]he element of race in cancer mortality [is] a matter of exceptional interest and importance."[39] His argument throughout the 1910s and 1920s was that blacks had been generally free of cancer under slavery, yet as their social conditions approached those of civilized whites so would the frequency of cancer among this race.[40]

Hoffman also stressed that racial "constitution" or anatomy, even if vaguely defined, was another factor affecting the incidence of cancer. In 1921 he examined clinical reports from the famed New Orleans Charity Hospital—an institution that traditionally admitted and treated patients regardless of color—for the decade 1909–19. These records showed that black women treated at Charity evidenced roughly the same number of uterine tumors as this hospital's white women patients. What did he mean by Negro? he asked his audience, the Columbia (S.C.) Medical Society, and how did race affect cancer incidence? Hoffman explained that mulattos had most likely a higher rate of cancer than "pure" blacks: "The term 'negro' for the present purpose is, of course, used in the generally accepted sense of the term, but if it were possible to separate the mixed-blood from those who are still relative pure-blood, I am inclined to think that the evidence would disclose a higher rate of cancer occurrence among those having a relatively large proportion of white intermixture."[41]

An important compendium of the presumably scientific, sociobiological, and medical literature supporting racialism was Robert W. Shufeldt's *America's Greatest Problem: The Negro* (1915).[42] A major in the United States army medical corps, Shufeldt's study contained extensive excerpts of anatomical and anthropological research he believed proved Negro inferiority. This research ranged from crude anthrometrics, "visual" evidence such as plates of photographs of black persons juxtaposed alongside those of apes, and evolutionist pronouncements, to clinical "reports" strewn with wild Negrophobic deductions. For example, Henry P. de Forest, a medical professor from New York quoted heavily by Shufeldt, asserted that "hospital records show that practically all male city Negroes indulge in promiscuous [behavior] and carry with them venereal disease."[43]

Shufeldt argued that civil equality and economic programs for blacks were only minor problems compared to the health peril created by the millions of freed Africans now concentrated in the United States and other Western countries: "The gravest problem to be faced in dealing with the . . . negro is not his or her industrial future or right to social equality with the white man or woman. It is the danger to the public of his or her contagiousness and infections from the standpoint of physical and moral disease."[44] The South Carolina physician, Robert Wilson, Jr., seconded Shufeldt, warning that "the negro is a public health problem of the highest importance can scarcely be gainsaid." Wilson cited a British counterpart, Sir Harry Johnston, who was considered an international authority on Negroes in the Western world.[45] Johnston characterized the Negro as "a hive of dangerous germs [who] perhaps has been the greatest disease-spreader among the other sub-species of *Homo sapiens.*"[46]

No matter how much rhetorical "fire and brimstone" health, government, and science authorities injected into their public warnings that blacks were a health menace, facts, statistics, and case studies would have to be marshaled to establish the scientific "validity" of their claims (the same, of course, held true for the opponents of such racialism). Because local government and medical examiner mortality reporting, public health survey techniques, and federal census enumeration of births and deaths were only just becoming standardized and expansive, clear patterns of disease, sickness, and mortality for blacks and Americans generally were pieced together from a variety of data.[47] What sufficed for health authorities seeking an immediate, comprehensive explanation for black health inferiority were the clinical impressions of southern physicians and public health workers.

The conceptualization throughout American medical circles of black health in the early twentieth century was shaped primarily by the medical academicians and practitioners of southern elite society for several reasons. Not only did about nine-tenths of blacks reside in the South at this time (1900), but northern medical leaders assumed that their southern white counterparts had effectively observed, diagnosed, and treated blacks throughout the two-century duration of slavery.[48] By World War I leading medical journals of the northern states and national medical organizations regularly published articles by southern medical researchers and public health workers that analyzed burdensome health traits alleged to be unique to Negroes. For example, in 1906 the *American Journal of Dermatology & Genito-Urinary Diseases* published "Racial Peculiarities: A Cause of the Prevalence of Syphilis in Negroes," authored by Daniel D. Quillian, an Athens, Georgia, physician.[49] In 1910 the American Medical Association's prestigious journal published studies by H. M. Folkes, a Mississippi physician, and Thomas W. Murrell, a Richmond physician, on "The Negro as a Health Problem" and "Syphilis and the American Negro: A Medico-Sociologic Study," respectively.[50]

The studies emerging from the early-twentieth-century South on disease patterns among blacks illustrated the profound distance that existed between southern medical sociology—for Durkheimian- •

like "social facts" or generalities were the substance of this medical thought—and the idea that dark-complexioned people suffered equally with others once afflicted. The studies also epitomized the broad utility of racialist conceptualizations of diseases throughout the emergent medical specialities. Indeed, this epidemic paradigm or collective sociomedical imperative that blacks were one with the causative agents of infectious diseases, holds a dominant place in the American medical community through the 1920s.

Quillian's treatise on syphilis, for instance, smoothly jumps from sociological opinion to clinical conclusions. He stresses that black Americans were natives of tropical and semitropical climates and thus have "sexual instincts developed to a very high degree." When these instincts combine with the black's "lax morals and indifference to virtue," according to Quillian, "the negro as a race is more prone to venereal disease than the white race." Quillian hops next into the "clinical" realm and back out to epidemiological generalization: "From personal observation I believe that sixty to seventy percent of the blacks in the South have either hereditary or acquired syphilis."[51]

A few years later Murrell's treatise on syphilis and blacks appeared in *JAMA*. The study's aim was to fill the "lack of statistical material on the subject and the consequent general ignorance" prevalent in the northern "white zones of our country." He argued that separate racial branches have entirely different evolutionary patterns. Thus, the "knowledge of syphilis as affecting the Caucasian, however profound, will not give one insight into the conditions confronting the negro."[52]

Murrell then proceeded to describe the sociological development of black Americans, stressing the widely held notion that as a result of the overthrow of slavery the health of blacks had been "crushed." To Murrell the direct physical effects of emancipation were now at the root of black ill-health. He exhorted that the black "was free indeed . . . free to get drunk with cheap political whiskey and to shiver in the cold[,] free never to bathe, and to sleep in hovels where God's sunlight and air could not penetrate—absolutely free to gratify his every sexual impulse; to be infected with every loathsome disase and to infect his ready and willing companions— and he did it—he did it all. The result is the negro of 1909, the negro of today."[53]

The black American in Murrell's view was now overcrowding the insane asylums and dying off rapidly. "He is, as a rule, but a sorry specimen," Murrell wrote, "for disease and dissipation have done their work only too well."[54] Also, according to Murrell's sociology of black communities, there was no sensitivity to health or morality among them: "Morality among these people is almost a joke . . . and venereal diseases are well-nigh universal." This researcher was so convinced of the black American's physical and social decadence, he could assert: "It is my honest belief that another fifty years will find an unsyphilitic negro a freak. . . ."[55]

Other medical racialism emanating from the South early in this century argued that members of the black race possessed exceptional immunities against common ailments. In 1911 a New Orleans physician who had treated about 600 patients for various forms of alcoholism concluded that "no quantity [of alcohol] which [a black] is able to assimilate has the power to produce on his brain and nervous system the profound disturbance commonly observed in the white race under like conditions."[56]

Modern readers should not underestimate the extent to which syphilis, along with TB, preoccupied the medical and popular mind at the turn of the century; hence, the strong scientific and popular demand for southern medical research on why the disease appeared epidemic among blacks. By 1905 syphilis was attributed to some 125 causes. Even the famed William Osler remarked that "the story of the search for the cause of syphilis is a tale to make the judicious grieve."[57] Since the fifteenth century, when new directions in medical philology, clinical observation, and pathological anatomy occurred in Western medicine, the syphilis dilemma had ensnared a dominant segment of the medical research community.[58]

Yet it was not until the middle of the nineteenth century that medical research was able to separate syphilis from gonorrhea, and 1905 when protozoologist Fritz Schaudinn and "syphilologist" Erich Hoffman unveiled the causal microorganism: the spirochete, *treponema pallidum*.[59] Still more research was necessary to sharpen diagnosis of syphilis, most notably Wassermann's (1906) and later Hinton's serological tests.[60] Finally, later in the twentieth century, the modern therapeutic phase or so-called antibiotic revolution was inaugurated by the likes of Ehrlich (the 1900s and 1910s); Fleming, Florey, and Chain (the 1920s and 1930s); and Mahoney (the 1940s).[61]

The ways that the medical community approached black Americans and syphilis during the twentieth-century antibiotic period was shaped largely by the limitations in earlier research tendencies. Three specific aspects of the preantibiotic phase of syphilis research formed the medical profession's strong predisposition for making and remaking the "syphilitic Negro" concept.[62] First, before the antibiotic period, the prevalence of syphilis was viewed broadly, through the lens of early international geography of epidemics. This world view of syphilis fit neatly with the continental or geographic concept of races that had been mapped primarily during the eighteenth and nineteenth centuries as Western imperial exploration and colonization expanded.[63] Indeed, prior to the early twentieth century, syphilis was approached as a devastating worldwide puzzle by the Western medical community and occupied a separate branch of the medical specialties. Typical medical textbooks were divided into separate sections for the major organ systems, which in turn were subdivided into subsections on congenital defects, infections, trauma, and tumors. Syphilis was listed as a separate section as well.[64]

Second, since the diagnosis of syphilis centered on the array of lesions it produced and was diagnosed mostly by dermatologists, the syphilis specialty, "syphilology," was interwoven with dermatology.[65] Third, early syphilology also centered on "congenital" syphilis; that is, syphilis contracted by an infant prior to birth.[66] In the early decades of this century, this form of syphilis was much more loosely defined than in its modern sense. Today it is known that congenital syphilis is acquired solely during the late weeks or months of interuterine development from an untreated infection in the mother.[67] But prior to World War II congenital syphilis was frequently classified as interchangeable with "hereditary syphilis": a form of the disease allegedly passed by genotypical traits of the parents and conceivably passable to third generation offspring.[68]

This universality of the syphilis threat, and its strong dermatological and (reputedly) hereditary features provided a major philosophical foundation for the tendency in modern America to interpret racially any black–white discrepancies in syphilis incidence and mortality. As data on syphilis rates began to build, and with the disease preoccupying increasing numbers of the nation's medical and public health community, the racialist response to the syphilis problem among blacks branched out.

One of the most active of the northern medical exponents of the racialist view was Dr. Howard Fox, a New York academician. Writing in an international dermatological and syphilological journal in 1912, Fox highlighted a new lesion phenomena to be added to several "dermatological peculiarities of the negro."[69] He described the abnormal frequency of "annular forms of the papular syphilide . . . in the negro race," and argued that this manifestation should be included with keloid, elephantiasis, and fibroma "as affections that are especially characteristic of the negro." It is noteworthy how Fox, like his southern adherents, easily drew conclusions about the black race generally from observations of a set of their specific patients. This is a classic error in epidemiological technique.[70] Observe this language to his readers: "[E]very one who has had occasion to see many cases of skin disease in the negro must have been impressed with the frequency and extent of the annular syphilide in the colored race."[71] In a later study, "Syphilis and the Negro," Fox again uses broad, racial phraseology: "The age at which infection occurs is apparently earlier in the American negro than in the white race, due to lower standards of morality." And, "[t]he severity of the disease is in general milder in the negro race."[72]

3

The medical and popular racialist explanations for the greater devastation among blacks from infectious diseases like syphilis and TB fueled an opposing intellectual movement. This counterinterpretation came from black physicians, as well as a small but growing community of social scientists and welfare workers. While many among the mainstream medical community accepted that racial susceptibility precluded effective treatment of blacks, the typical black general practitioner refused to give much time to this issue. In addition, the small cluster of the more educated, research-oriented black physicians, conducted clinical studies to refute the racialist position at every opportunity. For example, Daniel Hale Williams, the black surgeon of international renown, published an article in 1900 on ovarian cysts in black women. The purpose of this study was "the refutation of the idea that had been almost universal among surgeons, that colored women did not have ovarian tumors."[73]

As for other blacks in the medical fields, they considered controversy over racial influence on disease susceptibilty an abstract conjecture of little relevance to the movement for better health and hygiene they were advancing. Typical black medical professionals knew they had little power to curtail racialism in elite medical circles. They concentrated instead on offering whatever resources they could to comfort the disease victims, at the same time remaining academically and politically active in their profession. John A. Kenney, the medical director of Tuskegee Institute, editor of the journal of the black physicians' National Medical Association (NMA), and a highly regarded professional leader throughout black America, summarized his colleagues' views in 1911. In "Health Problems of the Negroes," which he wrote for the *Annals of the American Academy of Political and Social Science,* Kenney cited their growing involvement "in the crusade against preventable diseases" as one of the most gratifying developments throughout black America.[74] In light of this expanding self-help movement, he found the race debate in medicine essentially worthless:

> In many places, without quibbling over such academic questions as whether the Negro is dying as rapidly as some other people, or whether there is some racial inherency productive of its high mortality, or whether it is due to environment, the race is realizing that its death-rate is high; that certain diseases are taking more than their toll of human life from its ranks, and that many of these diseases are preventable. With this realization, many Negroes have set to work to improve their living conditions and reduce mortality.[75]

Similar denunciation of the racial susceptibility debate was made a few years later by another eminent black physician and professional figure, Charles V. Roman. A president of the NMA and professor at Meharry Medical School, Roman's ponderous book, *American Civilization and The Negro—The Afro-American in Relation to National Progress* (1916) was largely an assault on the racialist and eugenics scholarship of the day. According to Roman, this presumably scientific literature always rendered blacks inferior. "In medicine," he wrote, "the Negro is alike blameworthy for anaphylaxis and immunity. If he is susceptible to disease (as tuberculosis), he is a weakling; if he is not susceptible (as hookworm), he is a menace." Roman's book then offered a procession of cultural achievements by his and other dark races, as a counter to "a conspiracy of silence in facts creditable to the race."[76]

In the social science community, phenotypical inferiority of the Negro race was one of the burning issues prior to World War I. The 1906 Atlanta University Conference for the Study of Negro Problems focused on "The Health and Physique of the Negro American." This conference's primary aim was to bring before the public and those "who are eagerly and often bitterly discussing race problems" the recent advances in "anthropological science."[77] The proceedings of the conference contained excerpts of essays and printed speeches by some of the nation's newly rising anthropological and sociological thinkers, such as Herbert A. Miller, Franz Boas, and Monroe N. Work, who contested the evolutionist idea of an amorphous, inferior Negro race.[78] It was the participants of this Atlanta conference who raised one of the earliest challenges to the scientific validity of Robert Bennett Bean's craniometry.[79] Miller summarized the thrust of the conference with the statement that only "until different races have had exactly the same history can any valid conclusion be drawn as to their relative psychophysical capacity if mere observation is used."[80]

Despite their confidence that the medical and public idea that blacks possessed greater racial susceptibility to communicable diseases would some day be discarded, black physicians faced extreme pressure from their larger professional community to curtail the devastation from these diseases. Kelly Miller, a nationally recognized black educator and polemicist (and from 1907 to 1919 dean of liberal arts at Howard University), repeatedly articulated the almost religious importance black professionals and civic leaders attributed to the every move of black physicians. In 1908 he wrote of the particular seriousness of "diseases of a pulmonary character" affecting black city-dwellers. Miller found black Americans constantly querying "[w]here is to be found deliverance from the effects of this scourge?"[81] He answered time and time again in his many speeches and published works that the black doctor would champion this effort: "[T]he Negro physician must treat every form of disease that human flesh is heir to."[82] Since, according to Miller, "[o]ne touch of disease [like TB] makes the whole world kin, and also kind," the black physician held national importance. Indeed, Kelly emphasized "during the entire history of the race on this continent, there has been no more striking indication of its capacity for self-reclamation and of its ability to maintain a professional class on the basis of scientific efficiency than the rise and success of the Negro physician."[83]

4

Most indicative of the divergent responses within the black and white southern communities to the infectious disease problems of blacks was the massive public health voluntarism that emerged throughout black urban communities. At the beginning of this century, black health professionals and civic leaders were painstakingly knitting together a network of small hospitals and infirmeries, as well as public-oriented professional associations, medical schools, and nurses' training facilities. By 1906 forty voluntary hospitals and smaller health centers had been established, some of which trained nurses, as well as five medical schools.[84] By 1912 the number of health care facilities had increased to sixty-five. Most of these institutions were located throughout the South.[85]

Also in the early 1900s there were already mass drives throughout the nation's black urban communities to build public health and
personal hygiene consciousness. Indeed, the medical facilities and
professional training institutions were generally viewed by both
black medical professionals and black communities as part of this
public health voluntarism.

The NMA, for instance, grew tremendously between 1904 and
1912 from fewer than 50 members to 521. This growth was a result
of the popularity of the NMA's goals to organize black physicians,
dentists, and pharmacists; it also would "insure progressiveness in
the profession," and "help improve living conditions among the
Negro people by teaching them the *simple rules of health.*"[86] The
black hospitals were also viewed primarily as an answer to the
urgent public health needs of black communities. As the prominent
NMA leader John A. Kenney wrote in 1912, "[a]nother element in the
work of improving the health of the Negroes is the rise of the Negro
hospitals." Even the journal of the NMA was intended more to raise
the public's consciousness of preventive health measures, than to
report specialized medical research and practice. John Kenney
emphasized this in his 1912 book *The Negro in Medicine.* The *JNMA*
"is especially devoted to the interests of Negro physicians, surgeons,
dentists and pharmacists;" he wrote, "but it is so planned and written
that it is of general interest to nurses, teachers, ministers, and any
intelligent laymen who are interested in the progress of the race."[87]

Even more important than the progressivism within the black
medical profession, and generally overlooked by American medical
history scholars, is the outpouring of public interest throughout educated sectors of black communities for any health campaigns or professional medical activities relating to TB, venereal disease, or other
major health problems plaguing these communities. At its national
meetings, the NMA had at least one public session "when subjects of
popular interest are discussed in simple language." Topics ranged
from the "cause, prevention and treatment of TB," to infant mortality
and "the proper care and feeding of infants." Kenney remarked that
these presentations were most popular and "have always been given
in crowded halls."[88]

In addition to lay activism connected with the NMA, organized
public health campaigns headed by local black churches, insurance
companies, and colleges emerged throughout the nation's black city
communities. In 1905 the Men's Sunday Club was organized in
Savannah, Georgia, which held regular meetings to address improving community health. About 200 people would usually attend to

hear local black physicians on health matters. According to its president, Monroe N. Work, the Club proved that "the gospel of health could be carried directly to the colored people and that they were ready to hear and to put into practice what was told to them."[89]

In 1908 the all-black Knights of Pythias established a bathhouse and sanitorium in Hot Springs, Arkansas, where, by 1911, thousands came for "water cure" treatments. A year later anti-TB leagues or campaigns were formed in Portsmouth, Norfolk, and Richmond, Virginia.[90] The far-reaching activities of the Richmond league were described as follows:

> The third Sunday in January, 1910 was observed as tuberculosis day. A sermon on tuberculosis was preached in nearly every colored church in Richmond, and literature bearing on the subject was distributed. . . . A registered nurse, as chairman, did very important work by affiliating with the city health authorities in hunting up tubercular patients and providing proper treatment. The committee divided the city into districts and nurses were assigned to each. . . . Food, clothing, medicine, and even fuel has been furnished for the sick. . . . [T]he membership of the league is about four hundred.[91]

During 1913 still another community health group emerged in Virginia, the Negro Organization Society of Virginia. Endorsed by the Virginia State Department of Health and local voluntary agencies and health bureaus, the Society according to one health official, "demonstrated the value of a popular periodic campaign for a general cleaning-up of homes, lots, fields, and the community at large in all parts of the state."[92]

In addition to public health campaigns, the lay black community provided enthusiastic financial and political support for their local black hospitals and nurses' training facility. Black women's clubs were especially involved in this area. One German overview of black life published in 1911 was impressed that there were about 100 "orphanages and asylums for widows, cripples and aged, founded by Negroes."[93]

By the mid-1910s the vigorous mutual interest of both lay blacks and black medical professionals in reducing the damage of infectious diseases, preventable infant illnesses, and unsanitary living conditions, was peaking. In fact, Booker T. Washington capitalized on the projects and public spirit generated by these earlier efforts, when he initiated the historic "Health Improvement Week" movement in 1915.[94] His idea became the Negro Health Week movement, a nationwide campaign centered at Tuskegee Institute. Each April black community leaders in education, health, and church affairs organized a program to increase public awareness of health problems and self-improvement measures for the school, home, and communities. The Negro Health Week movement gained increasing public support throughout the 1920s and 1930s including assistance of the United States Public Health Service.[95]

Although this early-twentieth-century black health movement provided the seed for community-based or "indigenous" black community health mobilization, it had fundamental weaknesses that limited its effectiveness in reducing major infectious diseases and health problems of black populations. The immediate shortcomings were the institutional and technical deficiencies of black hospitals. Most of the pre–World War I black hospitals were relatively small, and focused on providing surgical services and opportunities for black physicians' and nurses' training, but not preventive health care programs. Physicians at these voluntary institutions, like many of their white counterparts across the nation, disdained contagious disease cases.[96]

As an example, the Perry Sanitorium in Kansas City, Missouri, had just twenty beds by 1911 and 90 percent of its cases were surgical. The twelve-bed Fair Haven Infirmary in Atlanta functioned primarily as a surgical site for local black physicians as well as white surgeons with black patients.[97] Through the 1930s the larger black hospitals in major cities—for example, Provident Hospital in Chicago, Mercy Hospital in Philadelphia, and Flint-Goodridge Hospital in New Orleans—received increasing support from major philanthropies. The overall function of these institutions, however, remained limited to what Michael M. Davis called the "educational enterprise."[98]

A second immediate barrier to expanding the early black health movement was that the southern medical establishment was unsupportive of both the black lay-inspired health institutions and the black medical professions' hospital and medical school projects. Public health officials occasionally endorsed ceremonial activities like the health week campaigns but not any sort of build-up of a permanent health care infrastructure for black communities; that is, an infrastructure with substantial revenues, ongoing screening and treatment programs and institutions, and capable black administrative leadership.

The chasm between the black community's voluntary health

network, and the larger medical profession and public health offi-
cialdom throughout the pre–World War I South was clearly evident
when the all-white Southern Medical Association convened in
Atlanta during November 1916. The major issue addressed at this
conference was the TB epidemic throughout the South's black community. A troubled audience of physicians, many of whom were
directors of TB sanitoriums, gathered to hear and discuss a study by
Dr. Martin E. Sloan, "The Urgent Need of Hospital Facilites for
Tuberculous Negroes." The head of the Fudowood Sanitorium in
Townson, Maryland, Sloan was considered one of the region's most
able authorities on TB treatment and care. Using vital statistics, information on TB facilities provided by the National Association for the
Study and Prevention of Tuberculosis, as well as his own question-
naire survey of twenty local anti-TB organizations throughout the
southern states, Sloan painted a grim outlook for the white South.
He cited government census data for Kentucky, Maryland, North
Carolina, and Virginia, the only southern states then in the registration area, which recorded nearly 4,900 deaths of blacks from TB in
1914. In southern cities he estimated that black mortality from TB
was three times that of whites, and in Baltimore alone 399 blacks
died from the disease during just the first seven months of 1916.[99]

Besides the high black mortality rate, Sloan cited two other factors that intensified the black TB crisis: the biological and sociological susceptibilty of blacks to TB, and the daily economic and social
interaction between whites and blacks that made the latter group a
deadly conduit of TB into the white community. "The susceptibility
of the Negro to tuberculosis is generally well known," he remarked,
"[a]dd to his inherited susceptibility an unusual fondness for alco-
holics and retarded mental development, and the host is prepared
for the ubiquitous and energetic tubercle bacillus."[100]

Sloan emphasized the sociological dimension of the TB crisis
posed by blacks, offering cold population statistics and menacing
examples of how infections could be transmitted during ordinary
contacts between black and whites. Roughly 8.8 million or 90 percent of the nation's blacks resided in the South. Of the several million black workers within the South, over 2.8 million were in the
agricultural sector; thus, they would "handle directly the [food] provisions of millions of consumers." Even worse than the relationship
of blacks to food production, according to Sloan, was "that the
Negro comes in closer contact with the white population than this,
for 368,124 were laundresses and laundrymen; 22,534 barbers and
hairdressers; 2,666 bartenders; 8,232 door boys and bell boys; 3,850

bootblacks; 8,428 butlers; 14,082 chambermaids; 92,301 charwomen and cleaners; 7,627 coachmen; 233,912 cooks; 11,119 nursemaids, ladies, maids and valets; 18,902 untrained nurses; 30,190 porters; 6,369 restaurant and lunch room keepers." Sloan cautioned he could give even more figures of similar exactness that graphically depicted how "the races are inter-dependent; the economic and health problems of one are inseparably interwoven with those of the other, and the solutions of the health problems of one must be to a great extent the solutions of the problems for the other."[101]

On the eve of World War I, southern public health authorities supported three different approaches to curtail the TB threat they believed was posed by the region's blacks. Some of the South's state legislatures were inspired to expand hospital facilities for black TB victims. Sloan encouraged all the southern states to follow suit by establishing at least one large central TB sanitorium, in Sloan's words, "arranged on a colony plan" for blacks having the disease in its early stage. Also, small hospitals in counties and cities had to be provided for the "hopeless and dying cases." To Sloan, public drives and disseminating literature were basically useless. "The Negro, as a rule, demands tangible (abstract) demonstrations to impress his plastic mind," and it is only within the walls of the hospital that blacks could learn the methods of TB management and prevention, while at the same time not be a source of infection to white and black contacts.[102]

Less extreme and costly than quasi-quarantine policy, a second approach advocated segregated divisions within existing hospitals treating TB victims. In Atlanta its 275-bed TB hospital had a separate section, formerly used for convicts, of 125 beds for black patients. But patient attendance was poor despite the fact that, according to Claude A. Smith, one of Atlanta's leading TB physicians, the city had "the most drastic [mandatory treatment] law for control of TB in the United States."[103] Generally TB victims, even those impoverished by their illness, loathed such hospitalization. And black tuberculars resisted particularly stays at white-operated TB facilities where they felt emotionally alienated.[104] "We couldn't work out the problem at all," according to Smith, "until finally one of the leading Negro churches, one of the 'ladies' aid societies of the Negro church" became involved to help convert the bunks to beds in the Negro section. While this support improved black attendance, Smith conceded that, by and large "they go right back to their relatives."[105]

The third approach stressed the need for employing black public health nurses. This appeared to be the cheapest and most effec-

tive means for increasing black patient attendance at local segregated facilities as well as preventive practices throughout the black
communities. R. L. Jones, a Nashville physician affiliated with a
county hospital that treated TB patients, vouched for this approach.
The county had both a TB bureau and four TB nurses. Jones noted
that "[t]wo of these are Negro nurses, and they can get at [blacks]
when white nurses can't." He cited a typical case when the hospital
director could not convince a black man with TB to admit himself to
the hospital: "One of the colored nurses called the doctor aside—she
was a very intelligent women—and as she expressed it, 'Doctor, let
me have him; he's afraid of you because you are a white man and
nobody can get anything out of him but a Negro.' And she got it
from him and got him into [our] hospital."[106]

　　Southern public health officials acknowledged that local voluntary black campaigns were enthusiastic and often yielded funds and
local publicity to fight TB. Yet, in this age when segregation of public accommodations was the norm, sharing resources and decision-
making expertise with lay or professional groups from local black
communities was another matter. As for the small black hospitals
and sanitoriums, these too were considered generally second-rate
institutions for use strictly by blacks.

　　In later decades individual southern states used all three
approaches, singly or in combination, to provide TB treatment and
control measures for black communities. In the context of the general social segregation throughout the pre–World War II South, this
usually meant that far less concrete, institutional treatment resources
(such as hospital beds) were developed for black TB victims.
Nonetheless, the belief in a causal connection of blackness with TB
gained a popularity and scientific respectability that widened as
urbanization of blacks throughout the South and the North
increased. Had American medicine not entered specialization—
which gives this profession the highest authority to dictate how the
medical practitioner, public health agency, and lay communities
should perceive and approach epidemics generally, and those
among blacks specifically—one southern physician's response to
Sloan's study would have prevailed even longer: "[t]he Negro is the
[TB] problem."[107]

Chapter 2

The Turn Toward Scientific Epidemiology: Black Migrations, World War I, and the New Clinical Order

The international military calamity of World War I created social upheaval at home that eventually toppled the sectional dam of southern medical race thought. Prior to the war, the authority of the South's medical elite on the issue of blacks and disease had shrouded the black American's health crisis from nationwide public view. But the war affected the issue of black health in profound ways: first, by bringing a huge population of generally able-bodied blacks into medical surveillance and treatment at Army recruitment centers and military installations; and second, by generating the economic context for the so-called Great (1917–19) and New (1923) Migrations of blacks out of the rural regions into the large industrial cities. This urbanization fundamentally disrupted the cultural environment and burdened the physical health of hundreds of thousands of formerly rural, southern black men, women, and children.

Immediately after World War I, improvement in health care became an overriding concern throughout black America. The fragmenting concentration of blacks in the rural South, the overflowing social problems within northern urban black communities that ensued, and the growing power of specialized medicine emerging primarily from the northeastern medical establishment, all drastically reoriented the momentum of the public health voluntarism of the prewar black community and medical profession. Social welfare and medical professionals working in the black community, along with their white supporters in philanthropy and private health agencies, looked increasingly to hospitals and clinics under the guidance of medical specialists to quell the health crises of the black masses. Before World War I the lay black health movement had been based on what Joseph Gusfield calls "traditionalism"—that is, neighbor groups and local organizations like the church as the central instrument for collective therapy campaigns.[1] But after the war such activism for black community health lost ground. Harried public health authorities, liberal white and black social welfare experts, medical specialists pursuing the microbiological aspects of disease, and influential philanthropists championing black medical training and disease control demonstrations, all began to overshadow this earlier lay black initiative.

The new post–World War I medical order centered increasingly on clinical specialization, identifying and trying to arrest microbiologic communicability, and promoting hospitalization over home care. In the first two decades of the century phenotypical racialism had consumed the medical and social welfare communities' perceptions and responses to the health problems of black Americans. Brown skin and African facial features had been an icon for susceptibility to bodily disease. But after World War I medical specialists gradually recognized the weaknesses in the construction of blanket, Negro race traits. The "multifactorial" epidemic paradigm defined by the growing specialized medical sector became the dominant force shaping the nation's government and charitable response to patterns of illness and disease among urban black Americans. The multifactorial idea-system also worked "inward," stimulating exchange in clinical discourse and professional meetings on racial and black health issues throughout the enlarging medical profession.

Specialized fields within medicine, public health, and sociology-anthropology generated essentially two multifactorial conceptualizations for explaining and approaching the black–white health differential: anatomic-geneticism and environmentalism. The adherents of the former conceptualization came from the earlier racialist or phenotypicalist trend and were primarily a mix of scientific, sociological, and medical experts focused in anatomy, physiology, pathology, microbiology, and population studies. They attempted to identify racial differences within the physiology or biochemical operations of the body and establish new sets of "physical" criteria for the races based upon a blend of physiology, static genetics, and anthropology. Their faith in genotypicalism most frequently derived from physical anthropology, which stressed blood-type groups to demarcate alleged races.

The environmentalist idea-system became most popular among public health authorities and infectious disease researchers, progressive social scientists and welfare workers, and philanthropists. All supported the expansion of public health care and the scientific and professional autonomy of medicine. Among their key ideas was that, while it may be theoretically possible to delineate races using certain phenotypical or genotypical criteria, black and white Americans had essentially similar inborn immunity and susceptibility to disease, and medical treatment had basically the same effectiveness on patients regardless of race. Race, then, was only one index to possible disease susceptibility.

Although radically distinct in their core etiological and sociological philosophies, both forms of the multifactorial paradigm encouraged more medical care for blacks, including early diagnosis campaigns and hospital treatment similar to that of whites. Prior to World War I the national medical community had no web of causal models upon which to assess national illness and disease patterns among black Americans. But the two conceptualizations of environmentalism and anatomic-geneticism encouraged medical and social welfare authorities to identify, experiment with, and expand professional therapeutic approaches to minimize excess black illness and mortality.

1

During World War I over 2,000,000 blacks were registered under the Selective Service Law, 300,000 of whom were drafted. The traditional practice of military medical authorities had been to segregate both medical personnel and patients by race. But during the war this policy was strained because the military initially did not have an adequate supply of black doctors and nurses sufficient for the tidal influx of black selectees.[2] In fact, one of the most urgent priorities in the eyes of the nation's chief black adviser to the War Department was the need for the nation to allow black nurses into the service "to look after sick and wounded soldiers who are now and soon will be facing shot and shell upon battlefields abroad."[3] Of the 380,000 blacks in the armed forces, 200,000 were organized into segregated units that saw service in France, while another 38,000 were concentrated in military camps in less urban states such as Kansas and Iowa.[4] In both scenarios black soldiers were far removed from the psychological support of their home communities with its black general-practice physicians and the traditional healing rendered by churches, respected elders, and musical institutions. Thus, it is not suprising that, to maintain the black troops morale, the War Department and Surgeon General quickly acquiesced to black advisers and implemented an all-Negro medical corps.[5]

The health consequences of World War I were apparently more severe for black military personnel than white, although in some

respects these blacks evinced health on par with or superior to that
of whites. The health exams of recruit populations and soldiers provided the nation's first national health survey.[6] They revealed the
military conflict took substantially more black lives in comparison to
whites. About 14.4 percent of the black troops died as compared to
6.3 percent of the white soldiers, an excess of 130 percent. Black
soldiers suffered more gunshot wounds, as well as the serious, so-
called "penetrating" and "perforating" wounds, and comminuted
fractures than their fellow white troop members. As for injury and
illness generally, black soldiers reported sick at a level 19 percent
higher than whites.[7]

Admission of black soldiers for treatment of TB ran about two
and one-half times higher than whites during World War I.[8] But TB
mortality for black and white troops serving in France was about
equal.[9] The most prevalent severe infectious disease striking black
military personnel was syphilis. Among the soldiers recruited for
World War I, the admission rate for this disease was 64.9 for black
soldiers per thousand compared to 12.6 for whites. Mortality attributed to syphilis in the Army was just .02 per thousand for whites but
.18 for blacks.[10]

Despite these discrepancies, other data on the health of black
troops reflected physical well-being generally equal to that of
whites. This pattern, startling to the white public and medical communities alike, was introduced in a study conducted by A. C. Love
and C. B. Davenport that was cited widely throughout the interwar
medical and social scientific community.[11] Love and Davenport
examined medical records of more than 13,000 black soldiers admitted on sick report. They concluded that blacks were more susceptible to "diseases of the lung and pleura" but less susceptible to diseases of the skin, mouth, and throat. The Love–Davenport study is
colored by generalizations such as: "[t]he negro teeth are naturally
resistant to the organism of tooth caries" and "[t]he nervous system
of uninfected negroes shows fewer cases of instability than that of
whites." In fact, their study concluded on the point that black soldiers possessed a bizarre physical prowess: "In many respects the
uninfected colored troops show themselves to be constitutionally
better physiological machines than the white men."[12]

One would expect this information disclosing healthy aspects
of the black military population to reduce the idea that disease
would extinguish black America. But the studies of the health of
black and white soldiers (no matter that they contained apparently
contradictory data) could not quiet the strong wave of racial deter-

minism emanating from the mainstream social scientific community at this time. For instance, studies of the military records on the physical conditions of blacks and whites were only a molehill compared to the avalanche of race research in the fields of psychology and "intelligence" testing. Thomas Gossett calls these mental tests of the 1910s and 1920s "the most powerful weapon of the racism of the period."[13] Such tests to demonstrate the inferiority of non-Nordic Europeans and most especially people of color were widely used. Thus, in this broader climate of scientific Nordicism, healthy patterns of black Army personnel were interpreted merely as reinforcing the idea that blacks were more the physical, but less the mental equal of white Americans.

In 1922 the popular magazine *Literary Digest* highlighted the Love–Davenport study along with similar comparative data published by the Metropolitan Life Insurance Company. The Metropolitan Life data also revealed that measles, scarlet fever, and diphtheria were apparently less prevalent among blacks. The *Digest* article, "Where Negroes Are Immune," emphasized the mystery of these apparent immunities and "racial traits and tendencies of the colored people." It concluded there was a phentoypical basis for these healthy patterns among blacks: the new data "suggested that the heavier pigmentation and more pronounced secretory activities of the sweat glands [of blacks] offer greater protection against these diseases than is found among whites."[14] The racialist interpretation of the health problems (or assets) of black military personnel blended well with a similar perception emerging among many health authorities at home regarding the mass diseases afflicting black civilians throughout the large cities.

The urban migration of hundreds of thousands black Americans peaked during 1917–19 and again in 1923. From 1910 to 1920 the total black population of New York, Chicago, Philadelphia, and Detroit expanded by approximately 750,000.[15] At the war's end, five cities had black populations in excess of 100,000: New York City, Chicago, Baltimore, Washington, and New Orleans. The black "cities within the cities" became more dense in the North, although the overall percentage of black residents in northern urban centers remained small. In a number of the largest southern cities, the proportion of black residents to general city populations was substantial. Blacks comprised over 45 percent of the population (as of 1920) in such cities as Charleston (47.5), Savannah (47.1), Montgomery (45.6), and Jacksonville (45.5).[16]

The urban black populations during the Great and New Migrations, sifted into hazardous living conditions and industrial work-places, experienced an intense decline in general health, most espe-cially in mortality and morbidity from infectious diseases and other preventable health problems such as maternal and childhood sick-nesses. Black mortality in the urban North stood in sharp contrast to that of the general white population as well as blacks of both urban and rural areas in southern states. In 1921 the death rate for blacks in mainly industrial New Jersey, New York, and Illinois was 19.5, 17.9, and 18.1 respectively; by contrast, black mortality rates in Mis-sissippi and Louisiana stood at 13.5 and 13.9.[17] Contemporary accounts by local social workers of the health conditions of migrants linked the health problems of blacks in the industrial North directly to congested, unheated, and unsanitary shelter, malnutrition, and industrial worklife. Infectious disease outbreaks and mortality, tracked largely by makeshift units within municipal public health agencies and social welfare centers, and, somewhat later, by insur-ance companies and the federal census bureau, also tended to strike most frequently black Americans working or residing in the urban industrial environment.

Investigators for the U.S. Department of Labor's Division of Negro Economics made a hasty national survey of the mass migra-tion of 1916–17. Municipal and state health data was skimpy, and the Division did not employ health experts on its survey team. Yet, using local health surveys, case records of social work agencies, and newspaper reports, the Division found illness rampant among many of the new migrant populations. According to one investigator, "[t]he most evident and pathetic phase of the friction and sacrifice accom-panying the movement from South to North has to do with the increase of sickness and death."[18]

The Division confirmed widespread pneumonia and other communicable diseases including "spike" epidemics of smallpox in several major cities. Philadelphia's assistant director of health discov-ered about 1,000 blacks suffering from pneumonia. Charity organiza-tions in Cincinnati and Newark also reported increased cases of ill-ness, "particularly pneumonia, and physicians universally gave similar reports."[19] In Pittsburgh, health authorities compared death certificates for seven months in 1917 with those of the same seven months in 1915. For the black population, pneumonia (lobar and bronchial) deaths increased from 64 in 1915 to 178 in 1917. Deaths from apoplexy also rose (from 9 to 20), as did those from nephritis (9 to 22) and heart disease (23 to 45), "indicating in all likelihood the effect of stress and strain of northern work and life."[20]

The outbreaks of smallpox were particularly troubling to northern health authorities. Pittsburgh, in 1917, and Philadelphia, that same year and again in 1923, were forced to implement mass vaccination campaigns throughout workcamps, mills, and city blocks filled with black migrant workers.[21] In Cleveland 330 smallpox cases were reported over a one-year period of 1916–17 by the city's board of health "traceable directly to the influx of southern Negroes." During 1925 Milwaukee experienced one of the most severe smallpox epidemics in its history. Lasting four months, 376 persons contracted the disease and 86 died. City sections occupied by poor blacks and Poles, and described by social workers as "overcrowded and unsanitary districts," were hit hardest by this epidemic.[22]

Urban blacks throughout the war and the 1920s were also experiencing extraordinarily high mortality from TB. Indeed, medical and government authorities throughout the 1920s viewed this disease as the most serious health problem confronting blacks. While the TB death rate among whites in both the North and South declined from 1920 to 1933, the rate among blacks in the North actually climbed upward from 1923 to 1926 and again between 1929 and 1930.[23] In Illinois, whose black populations throughout the northern stretch of its massive industrial centers grew profoundly from the mass migrations, the annual statewide TB death rate for blacks averaged 323 per 100,000 from 1922 to 1925 compared to 71 for whites.[24]

The devastation that TB wrought on urban black populations came into bold focus as local public health authorities studied more deeply their local mortality records. In 1927 Isadore S. Falk, a rising figure in public health care research and national health policy, directed a special survey of TB in Chicago. The surveyors had been charged to identify as specifically as possible this disease's citywide impact by race, sex, age, and time-of-year. The study disclosed that TB ranked as the city's third leading killer in 1920 but dropped to fifth six years later. Although the death rate for whites from pulmonary TB had declined, excessive black deaths had caused citywide rates from this form of TB to rise during 1922 to 1927. Among the Falk survey's most shocking findings was that TB death rates for the city's black children under the age of 12 were ten to twenty times higher than whites in the same age range. In its summary, the survey emphasized as its most important finding: "In 1926, 41.05 percent of the total deaths of children under 11 years of age were among Negroes who composed 3 percent of the total population in this group."[25]

As mentioned previously, tracking and explaining the TB

scourge among the nation's blacks, along with this group's high venereal disease rates, posed one of the most complicated epidemio-logical tasks to the nation's public health officials and medical profes-sion. Not only were TB and syphilis screening and treatment facilities sparse for blacks, but these diseases by their nature did not yield immediate, clear symptoms. The intricate testing and case-finding dif-ficulties posed by syphilis, which we examine in Chapters 4 and 5, would become the central objective of federal public health cam-paigns as the Depression unfolded. As for TB, following infection the risk of developing clinical TB varies immensely; moreover, the "lag time" between initial infection and the appearance of demonstrable sickness may vary from a few weeks to decades.[26] General medical opinion now is that infection usually requires close exposure to an infectious case over a prolonged period of time. This may explain why mortality rates from this disease rose markedly during the latter years of the mass migrations; when black migrant populations endured extensive stays in congested, cold housing conditions.

During the spring, fall, and winter of 1918–19 the great influen-za pandemic struck the United States. It killed approximately 500,000 or 0.5 percent of the nation's population.[27] Like TB, influenza deaths among blacks ran askew of the national patterns for whites. In late 1919 Wade Hampton Frost, one of the nation's premier epidemiolo-gists, undertook a survey for the Public Health Service of the influenza incidence in ten cities having populations ranging from 25,000 to 600,000. Surprisingly, he found incidence rates for blacks, even when adjusted for sex and age distribution, consistently lower than those of whites.[28] There was even some evidence that among males ranging from twenty to fifty-five years old and females twenty to forty-five, the influenza mortality rate for blacks actually declined during the pandemic. Moreover, a study of influenza mortality in Chicago found deaths among the city's blacks had been significantly lower than its whites.[29]

These patterns perplexed many medical authorities who had long believed that blacks were particularly susceptible to respiratory diseases.[30] As Frost remarked, "[t]his relatively low [influenza] inci-dence in the colored race is quite contrary to what would have been expected *a priori* in view of the facts that the death rate from pneu-monia and influenza is normally higher in the colored than in the white."[31] In any case, the sharp jump in deaths among urban blacks shortly following the year of the influenza pandemic may have reflected recording errors in the early reporting on influenza mortali-ty for blacks.

In addition to discrepant death rates from major infectious diseases, maternal and infant mortality rates for blacks shot upward during this period of intense population shifts and industrial poverty. The census data for 1923 revealed that birthing-related deaths were considerably more common for black mothers in industrializing states like Kentucky than in a more rural deep South state like Mississippi. That year black maternal mortality in Kentucky reached 15.4 per 1,000 compared to 5.4 for whites; the comparable Mississippi rates were 10.9 and 6.6.[32]

High infant death rates also clustered in the urban centers where black resettlement had been the heaviest. An overview of this problem by Forrester B. Washington, the head of the Philadelphia Armstrong Association (Urban League), placed the national infant mortality rates for blacks in 1922 at 110 compared to 73 for whites. He found the excess black infant death rates were greatest and even increasing in the major cities such as New York City, Baltimore, Detroit, and Washington. In 1924 infant mortality in Baltimore reached 191 for blacks while the white rate stood at 78; in Detroit these rates were 119 and 76; while in Kansas City (Mo.), 155 to 78.[33]

Health and welfare authorities cited major infectious diseases, malnourishment, inadequate child health screening, and poor pre- and postnatal care as the primary causes for the greater proportion of maternal and infant deaths among blacks. By 1926 TB, syphilis, and pneumonia caused 29 percent of all infant deaths among blacks, compared to only 7 percent of the white infant deaths.[34] A year or two earlier, a child health expert formerly involved with the U.S. Children's Bureau studied weights and diets of approximately 167,000 white children and 5,000 black children. He concluded the latter group was most frequently underweight and poorly nourished.[35] As for child health services, the situation was desperate in most cities with substantial black populations; as Forrester Washington wrote: "There is unequal application of educational and remedial [health] measures which is shown, for instance, in the denial of hospitalization, and the failure in the cities where there are separate schools, to carry on the same type of health work in the Negro schools as in the whites schools."[36]

2

Outside the edges of the black populations reached by local health surveys and vaccination campaigns, thousands of other black city-dwellers lived anonymously in deplorable housing and sanitation, and masses of them labored in the more dangerous jobs at heavy industry worksites. One 1919 study of 41 recent migrant families living in Chicago found 39 living in single rooms. An investigator for the Division of Negro Economics cited two cases as "typical" which would "help to visualize the problem." The first concerned a Georgia farmer who arrived in Pittsburgh with his wife and eight children:

> A few weeks after his arrival all of the children were taken sick, and two of them, 11 and 6 years old, died of pneumonia. Because of the contagion the man was isolated at home for eight weeks. His physician said the death of the children was due to the overcrowded condition of the house. The man received no charity and the money he had saved went to doctor bills.[37]

The other case involved a woman who after having come to Chicago a few months earlier, found herself in this disastrous predicament:

> Mrs. E. H. [has] three children, the oldest of whom is 5 years of age. She occupies one small damp room. Since there is no gas in the house, a red-hot stove serves to heat the water for the washing by which she supports the family. The water supply of the house is in the street. All the children were sick at the time of the visit; one had pneumonia.[38]

In addition to high frequency of disease, injury, and inadequate living conditions facing black migrants, these city-dwellers also suffered alienation from city cultural life and outright racial violence in their new northern urban environments. There can be little doubt of the significant physical and social psychological damage caused to urban blacks (and whites) by the wave of racial riots during the notorious "Red Summer" of 1919. Called by Franklin and Moss "the greatest period of interracial strife the nation had ever witnessed," during these months Chicago, Omaha, Knoxville, and other cities, North and South, were scenes of grisly street violence directed against blacks. In the Chicago riot 23 blacks and 15 whites were killed, and 342 blacks and 178 whites were injured. Also, thousands of blacks were dislocated due to strife. "More than 1,000 families, mostly Negro," according to Franklin and Moss, "were homeless due to the burnings and general destruction of property."[39] During 1919 one of the nation's most reputable public health authorities, C.-E. A. Winslow, responded to this urban violence when he told the National Conference of Social Work, "[t]he war for political righteousness between the nations threatens to give place to a war for social readjustment within the nations—a war almost as bitter as the first and far more complex and more difficult to comprehend."[40]

Race riots continued during the following few years, the most destructive occurring in Tulsa during 1921 in which at least 21 blacks and 9 whites were killed and several hundred blacks injured. In the older southeastern cities, where black populations were already heavy, black and white violence intensified and took a different form. Black contacts with local police frequently proved fatal as homicide became a serious public health concern for local authorities. In 1921 and 1922, J. J. Durrett, physician and superintendent of the Memphis department of health, and W. G. Stromquist, sanitary engineer of that department, responded to their mayor's alarm over an apparent plethora of killings and accidental deaths in their city during 1921. The two developed a public health survey of violent and accidental deaths novel for its meticulousness and broad geographical scope. Their contacts, first with the local coroners, police departments, and criminal court clerks offices, were supplemented with information they obtained from undertakers who had handled bodies of victims. In order to determine whether the situation they discovered in Memphis was unique, they expanded their study to Atlanta, Birmingham and New Orleans, traveling to similar offices in these cities.[41]

Although it was expected that the black homicide rate would be high, what surprised Durrett and Stromquist was the great proportion of intraracial murders as well as deaths of black males at the hands of police officers. A total of 739 homicides occurred in the four cities surveyed, 520 blacks and 219 whites (see Figure 2.1). The black homicide ratio was 2.4 to 1, while the black–white population ratio equalled 2.2 whites for every 1 black. Durrett and Stromquist could not identify the cause of about 40 percent of the homicides they counted because in these cases the death or fatal wound took place outside the cities' limits. The other homicides were attributed to domestic or love affairs (20 percent), altercations (8.8), robberies (7.7), deaths involving police actions (6.6), alcohol-related actions (5), and gambling and business-related disputes (4.8). While police-action and interracial homicides were only a small proportion of the total deaths, of 70 blacks killed by whites in the four cities during 1921–22, 42 were committed by police officers

FIGURE 2.1

Homicide Victims and Perpetrators, by Race and Sex: Atlanta, Birmingham, Memphis, and New Orleans—1921–1922

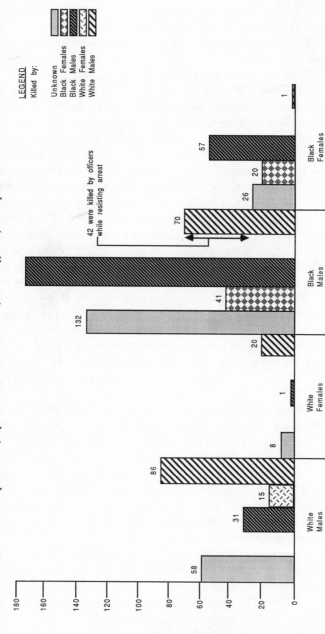

Source: J. J. Durrett and W. G. Stromquist, *A Study of Violent Deaths Registered in Atlanta, Birmingham, Memphis, and New Orleans for the Years 1921 and 1922* (Memphis: Department of Health, City of Memphis, [1923]) Alabama State Library, Birmingham, Alabama.

on grounds that these blacks had "resisted arrest."[42]

Nationally, homicide rates of urban blacks climbed steeply from the 1915–19 period (90 per 100,000 on average per year), to 1920–24 (103.5 per 100,000), and again from 1925–30 (109 per 100,000). This rising wave of homicides among the nation's blacks reflected both the complex effects of urbanization and poverty, as well as the overall youthful demographic makeup of the black American population. As leading present-day epidemiologists emphasize, in populations shifting from peasant to industrial contexts many "forms of violent death are intimately linked with the customary behaviour of young men, and the values and innovations of industrial society."[43] But during the interwar period, social researchers found racial discord contributed significantly to deaths of blacks during police encounters. "Why is the rate of homicide among Negroes so high?" Kenneth Barnhart, an Urban League researcher wrote in a 1930 study on the matter, "[a]pparently one reason is because so many Negroes are shot by policmen for 'resisting arrest.'" Barnhart found the pattern of police-related killings of blacks especially strong throughout the southern cities where many police officers were poorly trained. Southern white police were virtually always exonerated in these deaths. "'[R]esisting arrest' ranged from actually drawing a weapon and attempting the life of the policeman, to being scared and running when the policeman yelled 'Halt.'" As for black-on-black homicides, Barnhart traced them to (1) disputes that could have been resolved had courts and legal services been more available to blacks and (2) alcohol-related encounters.[44]

In 1925 Charles S. Johnson, the widely respected Urban League and Fisk University sociologist, conveyed the essence of the social, interpersonal upheavel experienced by the new urban black migrant. "In ten years," Johnson emphasized, "Negroes have been actually transplanted from one culture to another." Rural morals had been replaced by urban distrust: "Where once there were personal and intimate relations, in which individuals were in contact at practically all points of their lives, there are now group relations in which the whole structure is broken up and reassorted, casting [city Negroes] in contact at only one or two points of their lives. The old controls are no longer expected to operate." Elise Johnson McDougald, a New York City teacher and social worker prominent in the black community, summed up the social psychological stirrings felt by black women now living in the depths of urban America in 1925. "We find the Negro woman, figuratively struck in the face daily by contempt from the world about her." "Within her soul, she knows little of peace and happiness," McDougald wrote, as black women fought to "rise above and conquer false attitudes."[46]

The national educational secretary for the southern-based Commission on Interracial Cooperation, Robert B. Eleazer, cited social psychological pressures as the most urgent problem of black migrants settling throughout the North and West. Eleazer found the legal system unable to contain the ascending scale of civil violence against urban blacks.[47] Summarizing the situation in the mid-1920s, Eleazer wrote: "In many industrial centers the incoming tides of Negro migration have developed serious situations, which still await solution." These conditions spanned the spectrum of social violence and ostracism: "Bombings and mob attacks on Negro property in Chicago, Detroit, and other centers; the emergence of the separate school question in Cleveland and Dayton; efforts to restrict Negro residential areas in city after city; street clashes in New York, Brooklyn, Philadelphia, Beverly, N.J.—these are unhappy manifestations of a spirit that the North did not realize it possessed."[48]

3

In this atmosphere of poverty, racial tension, and rapid change, the new black urban dwellers, no matter how ill from disease or injury, had little trust for white medical caregivers. Moreover, treatment arrangements in hospitals usually reflected the segregation of the larger city community. Generally, blacks had been admitted to city hospitals dating back to the nineteenth century. But if they composed a large portion of a city section's population and went to a nearby white-controlled hospital, they were usually placed in segregated wards. In his study of urban hospitals, Harry F. Dowling writes that in Baltimore's city hospital, for example, "[d]octors and nurses were drawn from the white population, although by 1927 one-third of the general hospital patients were black."[49]

Conditions that developed in Philadelphia were just as bad according to a 1930s survey by two health activists, Virginia M. Alexander, a black physician, and George E. Simpson, a sociologist. Within this city's three municipal hospitals, black patients—about one-half the patients at the largest of these institutions, Philadelphia General—were shunted to separate wards or clinics. Moreover, among the appoximately 200 physicians, 50 interns and residents, and 600 graduate and student nurses that formed the personnel of these hospitals, "not a Negro physician, student nurse, or graduate nurse is admitted in any professional capacity to any of these three city institutions." As late as 1935, Alexander and Simpson wrote, "No influence, political, civic, racial, philanthropic, religious, or otherwise, has been able to alter this situation."[50]

In some cities black medical, welfare, and lay leaders scorned conditions in which black patients were treated by all-white medical staffs. Thus, a few municipalities maintained separate black hospitals. St. Louis and Kansas City (Mo.) had such hospitals. New York City's Harlem Hospital became predominantly black during the interwar decades.[51] By the late 1920s national philanthropic groups involved in black community projects joined with black health activists to campaign among other city administrations for separate black hospitals, as well as to build a separate network of black general physicians and community nurses. Edwin R. Embree, president of the Julius Rosenwald Fund, described the rationale for this all-black hospital movement bluntly:

> In 1928 there was little in the way of hospital facilities for Negroes. There were a few Negro hospitals of acceptable standard but not nearly enough to care for the colored population. Most general hospitals, both North and South, refused to admit Negroes. The few which did usually provided beds in special charity wards. . . . The vast majority [of blacks], even if they could afford it, either had no hospital to enter or could not hope to find one with facilities comparable to those available to the white population. Often there were only a few beds in a couple of dingy basement rooms.[52]

City social workers during the migration periods described their inability to get working-class blacks to shun their folk health practices and spiritualism, and submit to the private or hospital physician's treatment. The popular culture of working-class blacks in both the North and South, for many generations prior to modern city life, had centered the healing powers on the respected elders, spiritualist prophets and churches, as well as lay midwives. But during the build-up of black urban migrant populations, social workers and medical authorities, black and white, usually misread the anthropological subtleties of this folk health tradition, complaining frequently about the lack of enthusiasm for physician services on the part of the black new migrants.[53]

Social investigators from the National Urban League called attention to the problem of conjuring in 1926 with a brief survey, "Superstition and Health." Citing physicians and health officers in

New York City, Charleston County (South Carolina), and Springfield, Illinois, the League blamed widespread superstition as one important reason for excessive mortality rates of blacks. In New York City, one young black physician advised the city's Health Department:

> Ignorance, cherished superstitions and false knowledge often govern Negroes in illnesses and hamper recoveries. Young Negroes show patriarchal obeisance to the aged—the aged are, in a large measure, fatalists. They are willing to leave all to whatever their fate may be, the fatalism that has cursed the Orient for centuries. This fatalism exasperates the physician, for it ties his hands and tends to nullify his efforts.[54]

Indeed, in later sections we note a central role played by black physicians, public health nurses, and welfare workers from the 1920s to current decades was breaking through the indigenous health system of the black working-class. Urban medical institutions and philanthropic health centers relied heavily on their black health professionals and social workers to close the broad cultural gap between white physicians and white-operated medical facilities, on the one hand, and black city-dwellers in need of health examinations and treatment, on the other.

4

The general profile of black American health and illness that filtered out of the nation's military, public health, and social welfare institutions during and immediately following World War I was distressing, indeed, but there were a few encouraging signs. The overall health of blacks, measured by national mortality rates, was improving.[55] Mortality among blacks from major infectious diseases, like that of the rest of nation, declined substantially from the prewar decades. The TB death rate for blacks, for instance, dropped from 446 per 100,000 in 1910 to 262 in 1920; pneumonia mortality, from 257 to 197; and heart diseases from 205 to 161 (see Table 2.1). Health and welfare authorities emphasized that these improving gross rates hid glaring racial discrepancies in specific mortality and illness categories found among black and subpopulations of specific regions. These general death rates also obscured surprising similarities in the specific health circumstances and outbreaks experienced by the "races." Puzzling findings we described earlier included black and white soldiers with equivalent TB death rates, higher pneumonia fatalities for blacks

TABLE 2.1

Leading Causes of Death among Nonwhites:
Rate per 100,000 in Successive Decades, 1910–40

	1910		1920		1930		1940	
	CAUSE OF DEATH	RATE	CAUSE OF DEATH	RATE	CAUSE OF DEATH	RATE	CAUSE OF DEATH	RATE
1.	Tuberculosis	445.5	Tuberculosis	262.4	Heart Disease	224.7	Heart Disease	247.7
2.	Pneumonia	256.9	Pneumonia	196.9	Tuberculosis	192.0	Tuberculosis	127.6
3.	Heart Disease	204.8	Heart Disease	160.7	Nephritis	138.7	Nephritis	124.3
4.	Diarrhea	147.1	Nephritis	111.1	Pneumonia	138.4	Intracranial Lesions	111.4
5.	Intracranial Lesions	102.3	Influenza	107.5	Intracranial Lesions	108.2	Pneumonia	92.4
6.	Accident	93.0	Intracranial Lesions	87.7	Accident	86.0	Cancer	78.2
7.	Cancer	54.0	Accident	78.2	Cancer	56.6	Accident	77.0
8.	Premature Birth	53.6	Diarrhea	71.4	Syphilis	52.5	Syphilis	54.1
9.	Bronchitis	36.5	Premature Death	53.6	Diarrhea	44.0	Premature Birth	37.4
10.	—	—	Cancer	48.5	Premature Birth	42.5	Homicide	33.2

Source: United States Bureau of the Census, *Vital Statistics Rates in the United States, 1900–1940* (1943), 12, 274–89.

but lower influenza deaths during the pandemic of 1918, and black urban migrant communities with a disproportionate array of deadly preventable disorders.

Throughout the later 1910s and 1920s the notion of a vocal cluster of southern white medical authorities that post-Emancipation blacks were racially (phenotypically) susceptible to infectious diseases like TB and syphilis still echoed strongly through much of the northern discourse on disease and American races. But there was also a new thrust in medical and public health research questioning this traditional construction. During the war and mass black migrations, hospital authorities and academics (primarily from the academic medical institutions in the Northeast) uncovered mixed clinical patterns among black patients. As a result, profound destabilization began to spread throughout the knowledge base of the nation's medical and social science communities. This new medical thought tended to explain the high infectious disease mortality among blacks "multifactorily"; that is, as a product of complex environmental factors such as living conditions, employment experiences, and diet, on the one hand, or anatomic and genotypical traits, on the other. By the end of the 1920s many public health experts even went so far as to argue that TB and other major infectious diseases appeared to strike people similarly, regardless of their racial identity, when subjected to identical environmental factors conducive to these diseases.

During the interwar decades the new multifactorial construction of race and disease itself split into two overlapping subparadigms. *Environmentalism* emphasized the social neutrality of infectious microbes, maintaining that immediate living conditions, employment experiences, diet, and availability of health care were the primary determinants for the variation in disease rates among blacks and whites.[56] *Anatomic-genetics* emerged from the evolutionary, hereditarian tradition and, following World War II, a synthesis of physiology and static genetics, and most recently, sociobiology.[57] It explained the black–white disease gap on the basis of fixed genetic or hereditary factors manifested by differences in constitutional or anatomical makeup and organ peculiarities, or disease immunity. Later proponents of anatomic-genetics would rally under a narrow epidemiology which fixed the primary cause for many diseases of individuals and their families on inheritance, while considering larger environmental factors as merely dependent variables.

The new multifactorial construction of epidemics striking the nation's urban blacks was from the beginning a complement of the ongoing, still substantial influence of racialism. Indeed, throughout the 1920s and even into the 1930s, a significant community of American social scientists and policy thinkers still believed that the social and health experiences of race groups were extensions of the particular biological traits of the races. Biological reductionism was strongly present, for instance, in 1925 when some of the nation's most prominent sociologists delivered papers at the American Sociological Society's conference. A central theme of the meeting was to explore the traditional connection between sociology and biology. Many participants emphasized the continued popularity throughout academic sociology of the biologist's creed that "sociology is merely a part of biology." At the conference, E. H. Sutherland enunciated the meeting's general premise: that "[M]ost sociologists . . . appropriate a considerable mass of biological materials for presentation in their books and lectures, and justify this procedure either by the similarity of the biological and sociological processes or by the importance of the biological processes as causes of the sociological processes."[58]

The race relations and health sociologists of the interwar period subscribing to biological-racial sociology advanced a Darwinian, hereditarian concept to interpret the mass migrations of blacks and the ill-health that attended such migrating populations. They explained the black urban migrations on a broad scale, as if part of an intercontinental evolutionary process, that would prove a destructive end for urban blacks. Black social scientists repeatedly criticized the lack of objectivity that biological sociology perpetuated. In 1925 economist Abram L. Harris published a stinging critique of a study by Grove S. Dow, one of the leading sociologists advocating the "biologic-determinist" or hereditarian intepretation of black American social problems. Harris called Dow's work "a classic example of the American student's proneness to separate for special treatment certain illusory *Negroid traits.*"[59] Such criticism, however, usually fell on deaf ears in the mainstream sociology community. Indeed, with racial violence pervading both American cities and the deep South, and the advance of the serological technique of blood-grouping that seemed revolutionary, these early sociobiologists were strengthened in their belief that genotypical traits were irrefutably both indicators and actual determinants of differing races. To these population biologists, static genetic race traits were the basis for differing black and white disease mortality patterns, as well as the bloody racial strife pervading American cities.

This genotypical component in racialist medical and sociological thought grew out of a forceful river of physical anthropology and serological studies opened by Karl Landersteiner around 1901. Landersteiner was a Viennese doctor who went on to become a Nobel laureate in the medicine or physiology category. Beginning around 1901, science historian Daniel Kevles explains, Landersteiner established that the blood of patients contained three different substances (isoagglutinins) that reacted to certain antibodies. He classified these patients' blood "A," "B," and "O"; and later, along with his co-researcher Philip Levine, added three more blood groups, "M," "N," and "MN."[60] During the war years and the 1920s it was discovered that these blood groups appeared to be inheritable in accord with Mendelian principles. Medical researchers, especially the Hirschfelds and Ottenberg, concluded from their early field surveys that phenotypical "races" or "nationalities" such as "Eskimos," "Turks," "Hindus," could be classified as discrete populations or expressions of their particular blood groups. The Hirschfelds called these blood group ratios the "Biochemical Race Index."[61]

Repeatedly, however, the blood-group race scheme was refuted vigorously by additional serological and anthropological research. Initially most devastating was the work of Ella F. Grove, an immunologist at Cornell Medical College–New York Hospital. In 1926 she discovered that the blood-group features of the Ainu, an isolated, presumably pure "race" of northern Japanese, differed markedly from those of Ainu living in different geographic regions. According to the Hirschfeld–Ottenberg index, the distribution of blood types should have been similar for all Ainu. Furthermore, assuming that the Hirschfeld–Ottenberg index was valid, the data from Grove's serological survey would make "it necessary to place these white-skinned, hairy people with peoples as unlike them as the Senegal Negroes, the Sumatra Chinese, the Annamese Malays, the Sulu Moros, and the Javans."[62] Additional research that employed a blood-group race index to establish an allegedly pure "Negro" race—linking genotypically the blacks of North and South America, and Africa into a kind of separate species—was also stingingly disproved by other studies that appeared during the interwar years.[63]

The new genotypical racialism, however, also had an evolutionary or *socio*biological aspect that added to its appeal and persistent influence in social scientific circles. The prominent American sociologists Edward Reuter and Samuel J. Holmes, for example, evaluated black urban migration on a grand, Darwinian scale. To Reuter the urban influx of blacks signaled but another phase in the black race's desperate struggle for physical survival. Reuter described the black migration phenomenon as an "effort of . . . selective migration" on the part of black Americans. "This remarkable migration of Negroes brought into these northern cities a large number of young, active, and relatively healthy Negroes" which improved the overall mortality and illness rates of urban black populations.[64] Extreme poverty and congested housing, however, often greeted these newcomers. Referring to clear evidence that the highest mortality rates for black Americans occurred in northern and western states in which in-migration was heaviest, Reuter wrote that "[t]he Negroes have fared poorly when settled in the cities."[65] He adduced that such discrepancies in social development and health between blacks and whites resulted as much from a "racial reference" as from economic or caste factors.[66]

During the interwar period, Samuel Holmes, a zoologist and human biologist (as well as sociologist), became one of the most influential of the eugenics scholars.[67] Over the course of the 1920s and 1930s, he also explained the health problems and decrepit living conditions of black migrants in social Darwinian terms, a prelude as it were to an ultimate struggle between white and black Americans for survival. "Altogether, Negro life in our large cities does not present a pleasant picture," he wrote of the growth of black urban populations. In Holmes's view, these harsh conditions actually "toughened" black urban dwellers for competition with whites:

> Negroes usually first gain a foothold in the most undesirable and unwholesome parts of the city, where they are brought into contact with the worst elements of the white population. . . . The fact that the Negroes occupy an economic and social status inferior to that of the whites will probably be a positive biological advantage. If carried beyond rather modest limits, prosperity, especially in urban populations, is commonly a prelude to extinction.[68]

In a slew of articles, later the bases for his magnum opus, *The Negro's Struggle For Survival* (1937), Holmes amassed an eclectic array of vital statistics, medical findings, and cartographic materials to buttress his forecast. Even southern sociologists of liberal bent shared his idea that black migration was bringing on a national interracial struggle for existence.[69]

Broader diffusion of and faith in scientific knowledge based on the inductive, experimental, or clinical style of observations, however, subdivided approaches more than harmonized them. Observations of black health conditions by specialty-oriented medical and social welfare advocates disclaimed as too abstract the Spencerian determinism and eugenics of social biologists like Reuter and Holmes. These new health experts were increasingly drawn to the method of clinical case management not sociological generalization, and built cautiously specific cross-racial health data. At the end of World War I, the picture of disease among black Americans had alarmed these professional communities. But by the mid- and late 1920s many medical and welfare investigators doubted that a fixed system of racial classification was the most genuinely scientific way to interpret and explain this picture. Because black American population and birth rates had increased significantly throughout World War I and the 1920s, and, because the general mortality indicators for blacks were showing improvement, growing numbers of medical and social welfare thinkers discounted, for instance, predictions that the black American would inevitably vanish. In their view, America had to, like it or not, accept the challenge of understanding and alleviating mass disease and illness of the black citizenry, North and South.

The most knowledgeable and influential white public health expert on mortality and health problems of black Americans during the interwar period was Louis I. Dublin, a health statistician and vice-president for the Metropolitan Life Insurance Company. On October 21, 1920 Dublin shook up the professional public health and sociology status quo with his address at the annual conference of the National Urban League in Newark. Drawing from records of Metropolitan's 1,750,000 black policyholders, he stated that generally the black death rate exceeded the white rate by sixty percent. White male and female life-expectancy was 46 and 52 years; for blacks, 37 and 38, respectively. But Dublin stressed that data on "the particular diseases and conditions causing these excessive rates of mortality" could be used to guide the development of effective preventive health campaigns, thereby, lowering black mortality substantially.[70]

According to Dublin, TB, infant mortality, chronic diseases (such as organic heart disease and Bright's disease), and homicide (among black males) were most responsible for the black–white mortality discrepancy. He then retraced how Metropolitan's welfare division discovered that specific public health measures among black policyholders and their families could reduce excess mortality caused by disease and infant illnesses. Around 1910 Metropolitan had initiated a program of health "conservation" for its policyholders. The program included free, home-based nursing services, health educational campaigns, as well as support for local and federal public health projects. In 1919 alone, the company's nursing service made nearly 1,500,000 home visits, about 13 percent among blacks, and distributed hundreds of thousands of pamphlets encouraging healthy life-styles and the benefits of proper maternal and general medical care.[71]

After ten years, Dublin and other Metropolitan officials concluded that, largely as a result of its public health program, mortality among both black and white policyholders had diminished significantly. Comparing 1911 and 1919 mortality, they saw that infectious disease death rates for infants among blacks dropped 63 percent (46 percent for whites), while TB death rates dropped 22 percent for blacks (32 for whites). "In fact," Dublin reported, "if the death rate of 1911 had continued during 1919, we should have paid claims on 27,000 more deaths than we actually did." He added that there was "a great need for a wider extension of the work I have described among colored people." Because blacks continued to die more frequently than whites from preventable causes, Dublin emphasized that "[t]he colored people can profit more from [such] conservation work than any other race."[72]

Charles Johnson recalled (in 1928) that by analyzing the effects of preventive health work and black mortality by specific disease and age categories, Dublin in his Newark address had boldly refuted the idea that blacks were becoming extinct because of the TB plague: "For sixty years phthisic decimation had been, by most white students, accepted as inevitable to constitutionally inferior bodies, and by Negroes uncritically refuted along with the allegedly scientific findings which helped to fix their social status." But Dublin, drawing on health records of some two million black policyholders, presented "cold, stark graphs and figures" demonstrating, for example, that general black infant mortality had declined substantially. These data, of course, were "resented" by the doomsayers on the prospects of black American health and survival.[73]

Among the other leading white health and welfare authorities concerned about black America's problems with major diseases was James A. Tobey, a prominent biologist, public health expert, and onetime administrator of the National Health Council. Tobey sounded warnings to the general public about the health implications of the growing urban black population. Writing for *Current History,* a national affairs periodical, in 1926, he stressed that although social equality of blacks and whites was not common, "they do come into close commercial and . . . civic contact." Echoing the black public health activists of the opening years of the century, Tobey cautioned that infections between these two races could readily occur. "Microbes have not yet adopted the color line," he stressed, "and, in spite of the social aloofness between white and negro, even the venereal diseases have been transmitted from one side of the line to the other." The high infectious disease rates lingering in black communities that had grown with the great "Northward Migration," Tobey emphasized, "must be considered . . . as an integral part of. . . . the national problem of the promotion of our public health."[74]

During the interwar years, probably the most influential strategists for the nation's large philanthropies involved in health and social welfare programs among the nation's blacks was Edwin R. Embree, head and leading social analyst of the Julius Rosenwald Fund. Embree also excoriated the view that blacks faced inescapable decimation from TB or other disease. During 1928 he wrote in the popular *Modern Hospital*, "However bad conditions are in given localities there is no evidence that the [black] group will die out or even diminish in number."[75] During his career overseeing national philanthropic projects throughout black communities, Embree maintained that progressive science, not race theory, could explain and eventually eliminate the black American's health problems. He had been most impressed by the nutrition research during the early decades of the century on metabolism and energy requirements by physiologists Lusk and Atwater and their followers, as well as the pellegra epidemiology of Goldberger.[76] "Studies in physiology and chemistry are giving information concerning glands and diet that have direct influence upon life and health," Embree wrote in an academic anthology on biology and racial welfare published in 1930. "[This is] information concerning wide tendencies in disease and death, in population growth and potential evolution."[77]

In the 1920s and the 1930s, clinical researchers connected mostly with northern urban medical institutions, along with the large urban black hospitals of Chicago, Washington (D.C.), Philadelphia, New Orleans, and New York, also generated increasingly accurate cross-racial health assessments because of the growth in available patient data. This new medical specialism was integral to the explosive spread and increased quality of medical services provided by urban hospitals and clinics.[78] Simultaneously public health authorities deepened their allegiance to multifactorial epidemiology, mobilizing during the 1920s a variety of "secondary," usually underfunded and understaffed health centers, clinics and hospital sections for black clientele.

Between the two world wars the transformation of racialism

into multifactorialism was subtle. This intellectual transformation came as the hospital-based physician's diagnostic and treatment experiences with hospitalized blacks (and whites) accumulated along with the growth in laboratory data tracing the etiology and therapy for major diseases within the spheres of microbiology, pathology, serology, and genetics. Many of the new urban medical specialists, anchored by pedagogic background to social Darwinism, did not attack the racialist paradigm directly but revised it incrementally. This approach was typified best by the research of Eugene L. Opie. A biologist and pathologist, Opie stood among the nation's most influential TB researchers, concentrating on clinical investigation of the racial immunity theory. From 1924 to 1936, Opie was a central figure at the famous TB treatment and research center, the Henry Phipps Institute (Philadelphia), and later at Cornell University Medical School and the Rockefeller Institute. Generally absorbed with exploring the connection between racial heredity and susceptibility to TB, Opie's contribution to pathology grew as he sought to determine the association between focal TB lesions (of lungs primarily) and acute miliary TB, and its significance to understanding the etiology and pathogenesis of various types of TB.[79]

As mentioned previously regarding the unity between dermatology and syphilology at the turn of the century, twentieth century clinicians and medical researchers have traditionally relied on cutaneous signs and lesions to classify and diagnose systems of disorders. Obtaining accurate morphologic diagnosis and classifying these eruptions by their medical significance was (and remains) crucial to both the physician, for identifying the general clinical crisis the patient faces, and to the clinical researcher. Cancers, sarcoidosis, lymphomas, connective tissue diseases: all were frequently recognizable by cutaneous findings.[80] Opie sought to help unravel a centuries-old puzzle to pathologists: Why did the infectious agent in TB cause focal lesions in some individuals but more diffuse lesions in others?[81] He believed that, based on his numerous studies involving laboratory examination and pathological classification of TB that "the frequency of various types of TB differs considerably in the white and negro [sic] races."[82]

Opie's exhaustive research was a major contribution to American anatomical and experimental pathology. But its overall influence within the fields of TB epidemiology and medical care policy aimed at controlling TB among American blacks and whites was essentially antienvironmentalist.[83] Throughout his career Opie proselytized among medical philanthropies and professional epidemiological societies to make research and therapy in the anatomic-genetics domain the governing objective for public health policy makers and philanthropists involved in alleviating the TB peril. To Opie, more funds should be spent on expanding laboratory research on constitutional and familial-hereditary factors and on institutional care that facilitated such research. He saw this research and treatment focus as an advanced form of epidemiology.[84] Opie's view was summed up in the mid-1920s as follows:

> Analysis of the mortality and morbidity of TB by race [consistently] reveals important differences. The high rates in Negroes are conspicuous. The relatively low economic level, poor housing, crowding and dietary deficiencies are believed by many to account for most of the difference in white and Negro rates, but other investigators [like myself] point to significant differences between the TB of the two races when the environmental conditions are identical. The latter group attribute the Negro's high rate in part to inherent constitutional susceptibility. In contrast there are certain elements of the white population which, regardless of the economic level, appear to display exceptionally high resistance to TB. Again constitutional factors may be concerned.[85]

As many leaders in medical-service philanthropy became intrigued by the idea that a biological association might lie beneath the black American's TB scourge, Opie received liberal sponsorship for his TB-race research.

During several months in 1928–29 Opie traveled to Jamaica to research TB epidemiological among blacks there, while other Phipps colleagues focused on Philadelphia's interracial population as well as black populations of other American regions. Charles J. Hatfield, the executive director of the Phipps Institute, explained the importance of Opie's study of TB and blacks in a letter (1929) to Michael M. Davis, then director of medical services for the Julius Rosenwald Fund: "It is our feeling that the . . . study of Negro Health in Philadelphia would supplement the investigation in Jamaica and would result in laying a scientific foundation for health programs for the Negro." Davis responded enthusiastically, "Opie's study in Jamaica . . . will be very interesting and helpful in the health program for Negroes, and I shall be glad to know the results."[86] By the mid-1930s Opie and his colleagues at the Phipps Institute had conducted more intense, wide-spanning research on "TB among

Negroes" than any other clinical research center in the nation.[87]

Other research of urban medical specialists on TB and blacks paralleled that of Phipps researchers, also encouraging the reformulation of racialist interpretations and approaches to black infectious disease problems. One of the most important studies based on new anatomical research was W. G. Smillie and D. L. Augustine's "Vital Capacity of the Negro Race" (1925).[88] Focusing on lung performance, these researchers intended to add more empirical data proving that phenotypical characteristics, in this case an anatomical characteristic, determined the higher rate of respiratory ailments among blacks.

Augustine and Smillie examined two interracial populations. One was a group of 6- to 16-year-olds in rural Alabama districts (539 whites and 397 blacks), the other consisted of inmates (60 white and 100 black) of a state prison workcamp in River Falls, Alabama. Both the children and adults of the study groups were selected because of their generally good health and absence of any infections (e.g., hookworm or malaria), obvious respiratory ailments or birth defects. These researchers believed the adult group was a particularly good sample because these blacks and whites had (presumably) equal health, living, and dietary conditions.[89] But they incorporated key methodological fallacies by the lax way they established the racial "purity" of the children and prison populations under study. The researchers determined the racial membership of their study group populations by visual (in effect, phenotypical) inspection, and merely lumped what they termed "mixed bloods" in with the black group. "Practically all the negro children were pure stock, but there were a few mixed bloods among the prisoners. It was impossible to determine the proportion of negro blood in these cases of mixed bloods, so we considered all persons with mixed bloods as negroes."[90] Yet, although the Negro sample group may or may not have been of "pure" Negro constitution, these two researchers pressed on.

Measurements in the Augustine–Smillie study were of weight, height, stem length, hemoglobin, and vital capacity. There were blood tests for the prisoners to rule out malaria carriers and fecal tests for the children to rule out hookworm infection. The study concluded that the vital capacity of whites corresponded with the normal measurements established in prior studies, "[b]ut the negroes, both males and females, in all age groups studied, showed a consistently and markedly lower vital capacity than whites." They approximated lung capacity to be about 15 to 20 percent lower in the black children compared to white children, and 25 to 35 percent lower in the black adults. "[W]e believe that low vital capacity is a racial character-istic, and that vital capacity standards applied to white people cannot be directly applied to the negro race." Curiously in their closing remarks, despite the substantial differences they noted Augustine and Smillie cautioned against drawing broader inferences. "There is a temptation to suggest that there may be a correlation between low vital capacity in negroes and their well known susceptibility to respi-ratory disease, particularly tuberculosis and pneumonia, but it is obvi-ous that we have no basis for such an assumption."[91] That these researchers add a caveat against what they have just essentially "proved" suggests their own skepticism and the new pressure pheno-typicalists were experiencing from growing evidence that surface anthropometric criteria (skin color, "build," hair, etc.) for race were fallacious.

Opie, Augustine, and Smillie had been intent on locating the explanation for higher black TB mortality through the filter of anato-my, which they believed magnified a distinctive Negro physical con-stitution. They were, then, continuing the path of phenotypicalist research opened years earlier by the likes of Matas, Love, and Dav-enport. We have seen, however, that outside medical circles racial-ism in sociology and physical anthropology based on what was orig-inally considered a revolutionary technique—blood-grouping—had become irreparably frayed. Furthermore, during the interwar decades, a growing network of medical specialists, particularly in the fields of syphilis and TB control, as well as maternity and infant care, and public health and welfare professionals, wore away the epistemological power of racialism within American medicine and social thought. They were emerging from the new link between urban hospitals and medical schools, on the one hand, and govern-ment-supported health programs and black medical resources, on the other. These physician-researchers and social welfare experts added new knowledge (or reframed traditional questions), proving the inextricable tie between unhealthy social context and higher dis-ease patterns of men, women and infants, black and white.

5

The changing racial and therapeutic philosophies of Henry Hazen, a syphilologist and dermatologist, and Henry R. M. Landis, a leading physician-researcher of TB and other so-called diseases of the chest, exemplified the growth in environmentalism. Before World War I, Hazen began a professorship in these specialities at the medical schools of Howard University and Georgetown University, as well as a clinical affiliation with Freedmen's Hospital (Washington, D.C.), one of the nation's leading black hospitals. These associations lasted through the 1930s, by which time Hazen had become an internationally recognized expert on syphilis among American blacks.

During the 1910s Hazen's medical treatises on the problem of syphilis among blacks followed strongly the orthodox racialism espoused by southern white medical researchers at that time. For instance, in his studies published in 1914 and 1919, he estimated that on the basis of individual case studies by the likes of Howard Fox, Quillian, and Murrell, as well as data on Army enlistees, syphilis rates among blacks were from 50 percent to 200 percent higher than among whites.[92] Hazen's explanation for the higher rates of syphilis among black Americans, however, undergoes an important transformation. In his early research, he explained the black–white syphilis discrepancy in terms of the racialist argument that among the "poorer class of negroes" of the post-Emancipation Era, social controls were virtually absent. "The prophylaxis of syphilis in the negro race is especially difficult," he wrote in his 1914 study "Syphilis and the Negro," "for it is impossible to persuade the poor variety of negro that sexual gratification is wrong, even when he is in the actively infectious stage. It is probable that sex hygiene lectures will not have the slightest effect on this type."[93]

In his 1919 textbook, Hazen still sounded much like his medical predecessors of Negro inferiority from a decade earlier. The medical professor blamed emancipation and the subsequent moral misbehavior of blacks for their higher syphilis rates. During slavery, according to Hazen, "the negro was usually well looked after by his master, for he was valuable property, just as a horse or a cow was." Following slavery, blacks, "never . . . educated as to how to protect either himself or his race," were forced to subsist in depressed material circumstances. "Whiskey and cocaine speedily levied their tolls upon him," wrote Hazen. "It is only surprising that the percentage of syphilitics among this unfortunate race is not much higher."[94] Historians like Brandt and Jones have shown that this highly distorted image of black social organization provided much of the rationale for the notorious Tuskegee Syphilis Study initiated in the latter 1920s.[95]

Throughout his research of the 1920s and 1930s, however, Hazen became agressively opposed to the tendency to make a racial link for disproportionately high rates of syphilis found in black populations. In his 1919 textbook he had only interspersed cautions against overgeneralizing about the causes for higher black syphilis rates: "Statistics on diseases in the negro are very meager, and on the subject of syphilis are almost entirely lacking."[96] But by the late 1920s Hazen denounced much of the medical literature on syphilis and black Americans for containing "a large number of guesses, and personal impressions as to the incidence . . . of syphilis . . . in the Negro." He encouraged researchers to draw from a variety of surveys in progress: individual hospital and clinical studies, patient censuses undertaken by the United States Public Health Service, and the syphilis-study "demonstration sites" throughout the South sponsored by the Julius Rosenwald Fund and Public Health Service. Hazen stressed that special focus should be on ascertaining the syphilis rates of the black professional class, as he sensed that syphilis prevalence among blacks was not uniform but inversely related to class status. By the mid-1930s, Hazen is emphasizing the benefits of preventive efforts especially among black potential mothers who, if infected, caused an increase in intrauterine and infant mortality from the disease.[97]

Henry R. M. Landis was another white physician-researcher, based in an urban academic medical center, whose work intensified uncertainty within medicine concerning the reasons for the racial differential in infectious disease-related mortality. Among the nation's most respected chest clinicians and TB authorities, he was also director of social services at the Henry Phipps Institute, staffed at this time by such esteemed researchers as Eugene Opie. Since the 1910s Landis maintained that developing clinics with black medical personnel was the only approach that local health centers could take to increase black attendance. He employed a black nurse and black physician; immediately, the Institute's black patient attendance began to expand. By the end of the 1920s Phipps operated several all-black clinics, each treating hundreds of black patients yearly.[98] Eventually the extensive case-finding resources and record-keeping at Phipps for both black and white patients, as well as its thousands of clinical case records became invaluable materials for investigating both the medical and sociological dimension of TB and related disease.[99]

Landis in his early clinical papers (of the 1900s and 1910s) had stressed the connection between TB and "dusty" manufacturing trades, such as granite-cutting, as well as housing congestion. These conditions were most conducive to airborne spread of tubercle bacilli in the form of droplets. But Landis also emphasized that the racial element was of paramount importance in controlling the spread of TB.[100] To him, the issue of whether blacks had attained natural immunity to TB, as well as the social position and behavior of blacks must be dominant concerns in any movement to curtail the propagation of this disease.

Although not so simplistic in their assessment of black community life as their southern counterparts, Landis and like-minded northern elite medical authorities still viewed black populations as a major vehicle for TB's spread, not as potential victims like other segments of city populations. In 1923 Landis delivered an address to a state medical society that epitomized the alarm and despair gripping northern medical circles considering the TB problems of blacks. His speech, "The Tuberculosis Problem and the Negro," detailed the TB threat that blacks posed to white populations of major northern cities like New York City and Philadelphia.[101] Landis stressed that TB death rates for black residents of these cities were running two and three times higher than those of whites despite the overall nationwide decline in TB mortality. To his thinking, black urban populations posed a threat to the health of their white neighbors, because the former could theoretically continuously reinfect the latter. "Tuberculosis continues to be a serious problem with [Negroes]," Landis remarked, "and because of their association with whites . . . as cooks, nurses, maids, [and] laundresses," blacks were a "menace to whites."[102] There was, of course, a serious flaw in Landis's logic. He characterized blacks as a major contagious factor in the spread of TB, a common aspect of racialist orthodoxy; yet he did not consider, for instance, that white employers could hypothetically infect a black household worker who could in turn infect his/her family.

An additional problem Landis focused on were the health practices of black city-dwellers. He believed that northern medical practitioners faced extreme difficulty in rooting out TB from urban black populations because of the unhealthy social tendencies of these blacks. Although not so simplistic in his criticism of black social life as his southern counterparts, medical authorities like Landis still emphasized that black newcomers who "crowded" into large northern cities had been socialized into docility under agricultural slavery, shielded from physicial degeneracy by the master class, and did not yet possess collectively the natural immunity to TB that many Euro-American city-dwellers had acquired over generations of urban living. True, massive local and state campaigns to prevent TB began around the turn of the century, but according to Landis, "[t]he influence it exerted on the Negro population has been almost nil." He attributed this to the failure of TB campaign organizations to reach into black communities or employ black public health nurses, but also to the blacks' "aversion to going to dispensaries and hosptials,"

as well as the tendency of the black community's own press to over-
look the TB crisis.[103]

Finally, on the question of natural immunity, Landis believed
that much of the nation's black population, like its Native American
Indians, had not had historic exposure to TB and, consequently, had
little collective natural immunity to virulent TB infection. The natural
immunity phenomena, then as now, is exceedingly difficult if not
impossible to verify. As mentioned earlier, present-day infectious disease experts stress that it is virtually impossible to distinguish initial
and subsequent infections in humans, much less establish probabili-
ties of reinfections according to racial groups.[104] Furthermore, as
emphasized throughout this book, a "racial group" is an invalid
pathogenic category. Even if it were true that many blacks (and
Native Americans) had not had historic exposure to TB, this lack of
exposure was not due to an antecedent "racial" factor, as racialists
and later geneticists argued, but to long-term common geographic
and social concentration of populations of these groups that may
have precluded exposure.[105]

Nonetheless, by emphasizing more the immediate, in the sense
of daily space and time, environmental factors that influenced the
spread of the disease, Landis and many other medical authorities
were implicitly attacking the "natural immunity" tenet central to the
racialist explanation for the high black (and Native American) TB
mortality. Landis and his colleagues were among the first in the
nation to insist that black medical professionals receive staff appointments at every TB treatment facility that had a large black clientele.
Black medical professionals were skilled and dedicated employees,
Landis stressed, as well as essential to building the trust and compliance of black patients necessary for effective treatment and prevention campaigns.

By 1923 the Institute employed six black nurses and three
black physicians in charge of clinical and social services at facilities
operated by the Institute. This black medical personnel was frequently provided by Mercy Hospital, one of the local black hospitals. Black patient attendance rose considerably. In 1922, 192 blacks
and 832 whites were treated at the Institute's chest clinic. At the
beginning of 1923, blacks made up 727 and whites 1,070 of the new
patients at this clinic. To protect the accuracy and quality of the
Institute's treatment and research at these clinics, Landis and his
coworkers stressed a thorough and detailed diagnosis and treatment
record for each patient. Consequently, Phipps staff became experts
in non-TB complications of TB as they frequently uncovered other

diseases, especially among patients with respiratory infections. As the number of non-TB ill diagnosed at Phipps facilities grew, the Institute expanded its services for blacks to include syphilis and maternity care clinics. By 1925 the Institute, along with a local academic hospital and welfare organizations, operated what Philadelphia municipal and medical leaders came to call the "Negro Health Bureau." This was a network of four clinics located in congested black neighborhoods and staffed by twelve black physicians and nine black nurses making extensive outreach home visits.[106]

The environmentalist paradigm also grew considerably stronger within the fields of pediatrics and child care. The early (modern) movement to make effective prenatal care available developed in 1912 under the auspices of the Woman's Municipal League of Boston. In the same year the federal government established the Children's Bureau. Also, by 1918 the Maternity Center Association of New York City founded a prenatal health center movement and became the model for numerous other communities throughout the nation.[107] In 1919 the American Child Association started publishing its Statistical Report on Infant Mortality. These reports made available a growing information base for municipal and national health authorities, who became increasingly persuaded that social and economic factors were the pivotal determinants for high infant death rates.[108] As the popularity of prenatal care centers and infant health programs grew, because of their effectiveness in lowering maternal and infant mortality, obstetricians joined in by endorsing and working in such services.[109]

In the mid-1920s, J. H. Mason Knox stressed the need for epidemiological analysis of the black child's health problems; that is, of the circumstances that seemed to bring on clinical infections in the first place. At this time Knox, a public health physician and professor at Johns Hopkins, stressed that "if the forward march of public health . . . is not to be retarded" not only must the health problems of blacks be studied and improved, "but the physical condition of the Negro child . . . need[s] more thorough investigation."[110]

Knox framed his exploration of the black child's health problems on three levels. First, he focused on the impact of the major infectious diseases—TB, syphilis, and pneumonia—on mortality of infants as opposed to general black populations. Second, he delineated infant illnesses such as ophthalmia neonatorum (serious conjunctivitis in the newborn) that resulted from infections carried by the mother. Third, he specified unwholesome environmental factors or "living conditions" that correlated firmly to higher infant mortality and morbidity levels. In his 1924 study of preschool children in rural Maryland, for instance, Knox established that rickets was about twice as prevalent among the black children under two years of age compared to white children of the same age group. The teeth of the older black children of this same study group, however, were healthier than those of the community's white children of similar ages.[111] Since rickets typically causes delayed dentition and malformed teeth, this finding threw doubt on the popular conception that black children were naturally more predisposed to rickets and the disease more destructive to the black child.[112]

This approach by Knox attested that a growing segment of the medical community was discovering that health problems of blacks were neither uniform nor racially induced, but developed in complex patterns determined by the health of the mother, the pre- and postnatal household environment, and the general standard of living. Eschewing the idea of inherited racial traits, Knox and his co-researcher Paul Zentai emphasized in 1926: "The excessive morbidity and mortality rates among Negro infants are due to conditions which are a menace to the whole population, white and black alike."[113]

The environmentalism of Knox was also underscored in the growing epidemiology of TB in childhood. The causes of childhood TB deaths had perplexed medical researchers for decades. Moreover, the high TB death rates among black children had been a particularly intense subissue within this larger TB research issue, and the still larger medical and sociological debate concerning racial versus social determinants in TB's spread. With a chronic infection such as TB, the body at no time produces immunity sufficient to preclude repeated attacks of clinical disease that could eventually kill. Thus, the exact chronology and proximate cause of lethal TB infection was difficult to ascertain. Through the 1920s it was widely believed that most children living in urban poverty had been exposed to TB before their mid-teens. But in 1928–29 Phipps Institute researchers surveyed several thousand apparently healthy black and white children in Philadelphia. They found virtually no difference in the exposure levels of the blacks compared to the whites, nor among this Phipps population when compared to those of poorer children sampled.[114] Gradually more medical and public health authorities agreed that mass testing for TB incidence was extremely complex, and that such controllable factors as unpasteurized milk, repeated exposure to highly infectious tuberculars in the household, and poverty significantly underlied high childhood TB mortality regardless of the child victim's race.[115]

The 1920s and 1930s witnessed the rise of a small cadre of black medical specialists who were also important contributors to theoretical and clinical movement against medical racialism. Although trapped within poorly endowed black medical schools and hospitals, they persistently lashed out at the idea of black constitutional inferiority. Holding early achievers such as Daniel Hale Williams and William Augustus Hinton as their idols, the interwar black medical specialists took repeated jabs at racialist orthodoxy with counterresearch and political agitation. Among this group were T. K. Lawless, a dermatologist and internationally trained specialist in ailments of the deeper skin; U. Conrad Vincent, the surgeon and urologist who devised a standard operation for varicocele (or enlargement of the veins); George Shropshear, among the first to employ sulfanilamide—a predecessor of sulfonamides, one of our century's antiinfection "wonder drugs"; Hildrus Poindexter, an expert on malaria control; Louis T. Wright, the outstanding surgeon; Virginia M. Alexander, public health physician; Harold West, a codiscoverer of an amino acid; May E. Chinn, cancer prevention expert; Charles Drew, surgeon who developed the plasma so effective it was utilized internationally during World War II; and Ernest Just, the world authority on the biology of the single cell.[116]

During the late 1920s several of this small but extraordinarily active core of black specialists had few academic channels for critiquing advocates of anatomic racialism. But they did carry much power throughout the nation's "black medical world"—the traditionally black medical schools, professional associations, and hospitals—as well as occasional consultants or part-time clinicians at big-city health departments. In addition to the steady stream of clinical research these leading black specialists contributed to their respective fields, many strove to invalidate and demystify racial-reductionist explanations for the higher disease and mortality rates of blacks via civil rights periodicals, the black press, and public addresses.

The racial views of Frederick L. Hoffman, chief statistician for the Prudential Life Insurance Company, were particularly unpopular among the new black medical activists. In 1926 Hoffman used the mass periodical of the National Urban League, *Opportunity*, to recount the black American's health progress since the time he had published his *Race Traits and Tendencies* about three decades earlier. He admitted black mortality rates, especially from pulmonary TB, had dropped radically as a result of "better wages, yielding better nutrition, shorter hours, yielding a larger measure of rest and recreation and last but not least, better working conditions involving a reduction in dust and an improvement in light and ventilation." But he did not discount the influence of a racial variable completely for the higher black death rates, and, further, blamed immoral social behavior of blacks for its higher rate of illegimate births and venereal disease.[117]

A few months later a public reply to Hoffman's commentary appeared by the prominent Chicago black physician and public health researcher, H. L. Harris, Jr. The Chicagoan blasted Hoffman's article as "an interesting example of the difference in treatment which a question affecting the Negro receives—even from a man who is trained to the objective scientific viewpoint." Harris called deceptive Hoffman's data that supposedly showed, although black mortality from pulmonary TB had declined in recent decades, that a large black–white differential would continue to prevail due to some sort of racial distinction. Harris pointed out that such interpretations did not take into account that blacks were only slowly obtaining adequate housing and safer working environments; hence, the excess black TB deaths. "There is no support for the theory [assumed by Hoffman] that the improvements in wages, working conditions and in light and ventilation have proceeded equally for whites and blacks," Harris wrote. In fact, Harris believed that the lower mortality from TB experienced by blacks was quite astounding since recently they had filled shoes in the gritty industrial workplaces, formerly worn by European immigrants whose numbers were now greatly curtailed by federal immigration cutbacks. "Negroes in large numbers," he stated, "have . . . exchanged the relatively healthful life of a rural environment and the easy, open life of the farm for the death dealing conditions of the factory and mill."[118]

Harris also wondered why health authorities like Hoffman did not try to compare the "present death rate from TB among the Negro unskilled workers in the steel mills, factories, mines, subways and similar fields with the death rate from TB among the immigrant whites who formally did this work." Finally, Harris emphasized that some of the general health establishment's data showing blacks had a high mortality from TB but much lower cancer mortality rates were due to mistaken judgments by black physicians who were not allowed to obtain advanced training on such matters. If the Negro physician, Harris commented, "sometimes confounds, through lack of sufficient case study, the wastings of TB and cancer, it is not at all strange."[119]

Among others who publicly denounced Hoffman's interpretation of black mortality rates throughout the late 1920s and 1930s was the nationally prominent New York City surgeon and NAACP board member Louis Wright. A gifted academic surgeon, he would author or coauthor nearly one hundred published studies in his specialty, Wright usually wielded his sharp criticism against public officials, philanthropists and hospital administrators he believed were furthering second-rate hospitals and professional positions for blacks in medicine.[120] But he also, particularly during the Depression decade, used the black press of major cities to blast any insinuations that the high syphilis rates and other epidemic diseases among blacks were due to the Negro's alleged racial susceptibility.[121]

Before World War I, blackness had been considered an icon for contagion and susceptibility. At that time most white medical researchers concerned with disease crises of blacks lacked a theoretical orientation beyond racialism to explain infectious disease epidemics among city blacks. But during the 1920s and into the 1930s, when the medical profession was winning great social autonomy, the more specialized medical and public health authorities identified innumerable other factors potentially underlying excess black mortality from disease. The rise of this scientific epidemiology, however, would have been impossible had it not been interwoven with the expanding grid of black medical professionals and public health workers. This community-based, black public health sector provided a crucial bridge. It connected the new clinical medicine, public health and philanthropy to the urban black masses—all within the context of the intensifying poverty and socioracial segmentation throughout American cities.

Chapter 3

Medicine's First Line of Defense: Building the Black Public Health Sector in the 1920s

At the end of World War I most black medical and welfare activists believed the nation was viewing excess black disease rates for the first time as a *national* medical, health and social issue, not a strictly southern, racial one. Their optimism had been nurtured by the skill and determination evidenced by both black soldiers and their medical personnel throughout the war, as well as the growing body of environmentalist medical and anthropological research.[1] Throughout the 1920s and early 1930s blacks in the health fields enthusiastically supported medical programs for blacks sponsored by local or national philanthropy and urban academic medical institutions, as well as government public health agencies and campaigns—even though most of them segregated or excluded altogether black professional staff, as well as divided wards and clinic hours by race. Black medical and social welfare activists thought greater clinical and social welfare investigation of the major diseases and other health problems afflicting the black poor would result in more municipal and charitiable services such as hospital beds, TB sanitoriums and outpatient clinics, as well as training opportunities for black doctors and nurses.

Prior to World War I, the gospel of personal hygiene and medically sound community health practices had been preached mainly by lay volunteers within black communities. By the end of the 1920s, however, instead of the lay civic sector, black health activists tended to be professionals: doctors, social workers, public health nurses. They staffed the initial health care programs for reducing disease in black communities sponsored by philanthropic medical and public health sectors. As these black health professionals became a "superstructure," that is, an unofficial network dispersed throughout the nation's black urban sections, they also heightened the authority

of the hospital and medical professions throughout these institutions'
black-community clientele.

1

Health care resources during the 1920s for urban black America
emerged in highly uneven rushes: first in city (and, in the rural
South, county) health departments, general hospital wards, and
neighborhood health centers, a few of which were black-staffed
facilities; and, finally, in public health campaigns and health demonstration sites located throughout the nation sponsored by the large
philanthropic foundations, especially the Julius Rosenwald Fund.
The small black hospitals, infirmeries and sanitoriums were important for the training of black physicians and nurses, but provided
treatment resources for only a tiny proportion of blacks, mainly in
the South and a few northern cities. Midian O. Bousfield, one of the
nation's most influential black physicians and adviser on black medical programs for the Rosenwald Fund, frankly summarized the
severe limitations of black hospitals and the physicians they served:

[T]here are about 125 known Negro hospitals of all sorts and
kinds in this country, most of which are totally inadequate.
Upon them falls the burden of such hospitalization as one-
tenth of the population of this country receives, and such
teaching as Negro doctors get. It must be borne in mind that
the over 6,600 white hospitals, [usually] do not receive Negro
patients and when they do, they do not admit Negro physicians
to practice.[2]

It was the large urban public hospitals, the vast majority of
which were white-controlled, as well as municipal and privately supported neighborhood health facilities in the major cities, that were
the primary resource for diagnostic and clinical treatment for urban
black America.[3] And it was the black public health professional who
increasingly served as the "first line of defense" for America's medical, government, and philanthropic authorities interested in controlling infectious disease within urban black communities.

Throughout American cities experiencing the influx of black
populations brought on by the Great and New Migrations, only a
small number of their municipalities or social welfare charities established health centers for black neighborhoods. Initially, health center
services for city blacks were in response to the high TB and, to a

lesser extent, syphilis rates found among local black communities. The facilities were designed to offer screening and outpatient treatment for TB or syphilis. Later, these specialized programs gained larger support, expanding into health mini-centers that offered a gamut of services: minor operations, prenatal and well-baby care, as well as TB and syphilis-related diagnosis and care.

Among the most notable urban black health centers with the initial purpose of stemming an infectious disease threat emerged in Norfolk (Virginia), Cincinnati, and Philadelphia. During World War I, Norfolk had functioned as a center for military and naval mobilization. The federal government was concerned that service personnel be protected from venereal disease. Already having one of the earliest and most successful black community-based TB clinics, municipal authorities of Norfolk established a black community center that included a venereal disease clinic operated by black phyicians, nurses, and social workers. By 1932, because of the local popularity of this clinic, the city of Norfolk opened a fully equipped public health clinic managed by black medical and social welfare personnel. It served not only black residents of this city, but also blacks living in rural regions ouside Norfolk and transient blacks.[4]

Another nationally recognized public health center for black city-dwellers was the Shoemaker Health Center in Cincinnati. Established in 1926 to serve the city's West End section, a black community of over 17,000 residents where disease mortality had been excessively high, the facility became a multipurpose health care, medical training, and social welfare resource. It was funded primarily by the local Community Chest and coordinated the health and welfare activism of both white and black groups throughout the city. To improve their professional expertise, seventeen black physicians and six dentists practicing in Cincinnati were allowed to rotate their services at Shoemaker. Their clinical work was overseen by the superintendent of the Cincinnati General Hospital and dean of the College of Medicine. Less than a year after its opening, Shoemaker had several hundred patients on its caseload receiving everything from minor surgery and dental care to general checkups during their visits.[5]

In Philadelphia, the Phipps Institute's medical facilities staffed by blacks expanded throughout the latter 1920s. By 1927 these facilities coordinated by the Institute, known as the Negro Health Bureau, employed twelve black doctors and ten black nurses. What initially was a project to employ a few black professionals as part of the Institute's efforts to reach black patients for TB examination and treatment now had become a network of four dispensaries for blacks. "As originally conceived the experiment had in mind tuberculosis only," Henry Landis wrote in the *Child Health Bulletin.* "Tuberculosis is still the major problem, but gradually other health activities have been added." These services included prenatal, infant and child care, and syphilis clinics.[6]

When compared with the size of each of these cities' poor black populations, numbering up to tens of thousands, these clinics amounted to only miniscule health care resources. But they were among the best the times had to offer to what American municipal leaders viewed as an exploding and TB-prone black city population. Aware of the value and scarcity of black medical personnel and facilities, it is not surprising a leading white clinician such as Landis campaigned in strong and ordinary languarge for the expansion of these facilities in public health and medical journals. In the *Ohio Medical Journal* and the *Child Health Bulletin,* for example, Landis implored the larger medical and political community to follow the Phipps example and set up auxiliary black clinics staffed by black medical professionals. "The negro is here to stay," he emphasized, "and [a]ny solution of the negro problem other than that which recognizes that he is to continue as a permanent part of our population is preposterous and not to be thought of. [O]nce this is realized it is obvious that one of the most helpful things we can do is to educate him along health lines." Finally, Landis urged the white American health care community to realize "[s]elf interest and our own protection argues for this, if no other reason."[7]

Besides separate dispensaries, some cities developed a network of TB control clinics, paying little attention to special needs of blacks in staffing their clinics. Black physicians termed such city TB programs "color blind" in the sense that black patients from around the city were routinely admitted if they came in on their own accord. This was the situation in Cleveland, which developed one of the most comprehensive public TB control programs in the nation. In 1911 this city established a bureau of tuberculosis, divided the city into five districts, and opened a dispensary in each of these districts. Because of the strong backing of the the local Anti-Tuberculosis League, and the fact that the city placed the direct jurdisdiction and coordination of TB control centers directly under the municipal health commissioners, the city was able to expand this network, extending services throughout much of Cleveland's black residential areas. By 1930 Cleveland had eight districts, each with a health station that focused on TB control and child hygiene. Most of these clinics were equipped with waiting, examination, and nurses' records rooms, while examination and treatment was coordinated on-site by at least one trained TB clinician. In all but one of the eight health districts new cases included blacks; although districts 2 and 8, located in largely black areas, received the bulk of the system's black patients.[8]

Despite this comprehensively planned TB-control system on paper, TB mortality for blacks remained high. In 1927 blacks were 34 percent of the 789 TB deaths in Cleveland; in 1928, they were 32 percent, although composing only about 5 percent of the city's total population. Most blacks receiving care at these clinics were already in the late stages of illness; and countless others throughout black Cleveland went without care altogether. In 1929 only 16 percent of the total TB cases throughout the city were black despite this group's high TB death rate. District officials blamed this in-treatment–to–death ratio on deficiencies both in their care system and within blacks themselves: "[It] suggests either differences in the completeness of reporting of cases as between the races, less adequate medical care for the colored population, or that the colored people are more susceptible and suffer from tuberculosis for a shorter period of time before death than do the white people. Doubtless all these factors prevail."[9]

In other urban areas, small segregated health centers were established with prevention of no specific disease in mind, but merely general walk-in care. In 1919 the Los Angeles County health department undertook a major initiative to develop health districts and health centers. To serve the black and Mexican-American residential sections, only a small, four-room center was built by the county near Monrovia.[10] Finally, many cities that had health center systems for white residents, acknowledged needs for additional health centers for its black citizens, but simply did not have them in place yet. Similar to the health care services that developed to reduce high TB mortality among urban black adults, child health services for blacks grew sporadically throughout American cities. Philadelphia Urban League official Forrester Washington, investigating this subject in 1925, found "in many sections of the country health work of any value for Negro children is conspicuous by its absence." Neither Baltimore nor Charleston, despite large black youth populations and some of the country's highest black infant mortality rates (191.6 and 213.7 deaths per 1,000 births, respectively), had any significant services for these populations. Throughout the North, Washington cited as typical Camden (N.J.) and Kansas City (Mo.), both with relatively high black infant death rates for this region (131 and 155, respectively), but still "cities which take little interest in the health of its Negro children" and "[e]ndless other instances could be pointed out."[11]

Despite the dismal general picture of child health services for black city-dwellers, there were several exceptions. New York City, Cincinnati, Philadelphia, Memphis, and Houston all had local child health programs making headway in alleviating this great need. In the Columbus Hill district, which had one of New York City's poorest black sections, the Association for the Improvement of the Condition of the Poor provided both prenatal and infant care clinics for black mothers. In Harlem during 1922 the New York Urban League and the New York Tuberculosis and Health Association headed the formation of the Harlem Tuberculosis and Health Committee. The Committee served as coordinator for a variety of organizations wishing to do health work in this section. As a result of the Committee's work, "[h]ealth propaganda is carried on daily instead of sporadically," Washington observed, "through lectures given in churches and schools and through permanent exhibitions." In addition to a child medical examination clinic, twelve black dentists voluntarily gave their services through a free dental clinic for black children run by the Committee. By 1928 about 365 examinations and 2,200 dental visits were being performed annually for Harlem children.[12]

In Cincinnati, modest child health services for blacks were at least a structured part of the municipality's allocation of funds from the Shepphard–Towner Bill. This city added two black nurses to the three it already employed for black health programs, as well as two clinics opened specifically for black children. In Philadelphia, the four black clinics of the so-called Negro Health Bureau run largely by the Phipps Institute and local civic welfare organizations, also provided some maternity and child services.[13]

Memphis and Houston were two southern cities with significant health programs for black children. The former city, with a population over one-third black, provided both pre- and postnatal clinics for mothers and their babies. Services included physical examinations, serological testing for syphilis, and infant care instruction. There was also one black nurse for each 3,000 black public school students to assure some modicum of preventive health care outside the community clinics. Black children in Houston received medical care as part of a threefold movement to reduce TB, syphilis, and infant mortality. These services were provided through a joint effort by the city's social service bureau, the Red Cross and the Houston Tuberculosis Hospital Association. Finally, a number of cities, including Dayton, Cincinnati, Philadelphia, Detroit, and Memphis, stationed black nurses full- or part-time in all-black public schools. A small number of county health departments throughout the South each employed a black nurse or two for child health work as well.[14]

2

The disparate spread or, all too often, absolute lack of health care resources throughout cities and rural countries with densely populated sections of blacks—*not* a strictly panicky response to high TB or syphilis levels among blacks—inspired the Julius Rosenwald Fund to initiate a broad-scale Negro health program. The Fund was created in 1917 and administered directly by its founder, the Chicago-based business leader Julius Rosenwald. From 1917 to 1927 the foundation's chief program was constructing public schools for blacks throughout the southern states. The results were impressive to the nation's white and black political and civic leadership: several thousand school buildings were completed in hundreds of southern counties. But in 1928 the Fund entered a fundamentally new period of its development. The foundation was enlarged into a diverse enterprise controlled by a board of trustees and full-time directors who operated the Fund's expanding programs. In addition to its public education campaign for blacks, the Fund now added projects in medical welfare, library services, social studies, and race relations activities. With an additional aim to expand the supply of black professionals, the Fund focused major attention on financing the development of black colleges and professionals.[15]

During this second phase of the Rosenwald Fund's work, Edwin Embree led the foundation and its health care program with the idea that "[t]he chief scourges [for blacks] were tuberculosis, syphilis, and maternal and infant mortality."[16] Embree and the Rosenwald Fund viewed the problems of infectious disease and infant and maternal deaths among blacks as inseparable from the need for an adequate supply of black medical personnel and separate clinics and hospitals. Indeed, the black health professional strata that emerged during the 1920s and 1930s was primarily a result of this program. The Fund's black health program was a three-prong development. First, demonstration projects in TB and syphilis investigation and treatment were funded in cooperation with the Public Health Service throughout sites primarily in the South. Second, the Fund assisted a small number of black hospitals (about a dozen or so annually) to serve as training centers for black interns, physicians, nurses, and hospital administrators, while at the same time operating clinical services especially needed by these hospitals' particular clientele. Finally, its black medical program sponsored the employment of black medical professionals by local public health departments, especially those throughout the South.[17]

The Rosenwald Fund assisted investigation of diseases seriously afflicting blacks to publicize, and partially meet, the need for the nation to build a black medical corps for and in the black American community. This was evident in both its private deliberations and public operations. In the Fund's minutes of 1929, the pragmatic meliorism behind its new devotion to the medical problems of blacks was set forth. It described current health services for blacks as "in general on a far lower level than for most other groups in the United States." Hospital and clinical resources "are entirely inadequate," according to the Fund, so the "situation requires that the Fund develop a health program among Negroes which is fairly broad in scope if really effective work is to be done in this field."[18]

There were deeply rooted social ideologies, complementary to the environmentalist epidemic paradigm, that also led the Rosenwald Fund into this policy of nurturing a separate black medical force and hospital network to train and treat black Americans. One social idea was *parallelism*, an approach to interracial social and political matters widespread throughout liberal philanthropic and political circles during this period. Similar to a then-popular sociological concept among academics and race leaders known as *biracial organization*, parallelism approached a city as circumscribing two multitiered class structures: one white, the other black, existing roughly side by side but with the white pyramid dominating the black one (see Figure 3.1). The nation's black communities had their own professional (upper), middle, and lower classes and, as such, needed its own supply of black physicians and medical care infrastructure. During the interwar period W. Lloyd Warner and E. Franklin Frazier, sociologists, and W. E. B. Du Bois, the international scholar-activist, for example, all enunciated some form of this general idea.[19]

Another factor that shaped the Rosenwald Fund's black health program was the increasing focus by the medical establishment on syphilis as the nation's major disease problem. Before World War I most syphilis cases were treated but not reported by private physicians. With the growth of public health agencies, however, the number of these cases multiplied each year, and so did the medical and public health community's consternation about the disease's spread.

FIGURE 3.1

Sociological Concept of Biracial Organization
in the United States

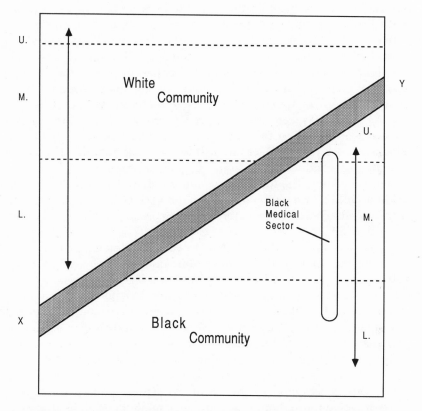

Source: Adapted from diagram in W. L. Warner, "American Caste and Class,"
American Journal of Sociology, 42, no. 2 (September 1936): 235.

Between 1919 and 1935 reported cases of syphilis rose steadily from
113.2 cases per 100,000 population in 1919 to 212.6 cases per
100,000 population in 1936.[20]

By the late 1920s the Fund trustees had divided its "Medical
Program for Negroes" into four areas: "studies and surveys," "health
problems," "Negro physicians and hospitals," and "Provident Hospital."[21] In the first two areas, the Fund took only a secondary role.
They anticipated that the United States Public Health Service would
lead in investigating the clinical and treatment aspects of both

syphilis and TB, while the black medical community would operate increasingly as the frontline caregivers throughout black American society.

Since World War I, well before the Rosenwald Fund joined efforts to alleviate health problems of the black community, concern with how and why the spread of syphilis differed in blacks and whites had been intensifying among federal researchers. It was one aspect of the government's larger interest in developing new, less painful and costly treatment, and preventive measures for this disease. In 1926 the United States Public Health Service tried to determine the scope of syphilis prevalence throughout the nation, adminstering a one-day census in twenty-five communities. The rate for whites was found to be 4.05 cases per 1,000 persons, while for blacks 7.2 per 1,000.[22] Over the next two years the Public Health Service helped conduct statistical investigations of syphilis in five major American clinics. The following year the Public Health Service assisted in establishing a national research network of five leading university syphilis clinics to monitor changing treatment approaches for this disease.[23]

To the Rosenwald Fund, however, the epidemic threat that syphilitic blacks posed to mainstream America compared to black tuberculars was decidedly less urgent. Fund workers envisioned that venereal disease among blacks, no matter how allegedly rampant, would remain within the nation's black communities. Moreover, massive research on the technical detection and treatment aspects of syphilis did not lie within the financial and operational means of the Fund. In 1929 the Rosenwald Fund threw its support behind the syphilis field research of Dr. Taliaferro Clark, the Public Health Service's officer assigned to the Fund. As James Jones has detailed, Clark traveled throughout the South, arranging the syphilis studies of the region's black communities. Assisting financially this activity for the Public Health Service was, to the Fund's heads, "[e]ncouraging studies in health problems peculiar to the Negro, such as the causes for higher death rates than among whites from tuberculosis, venereal diseases and infant mortality."[24] While the Fund supported a TB study and demonstration site in a southern rural region of Tennessee as well as a black sanitorium in Arkansas, it mainly deferred the TB concern to the Public Health Service and the National Tuberculosis Association.[25]

The leaders of the Rosenwald Fund believed the only long-term solution to the other health problems of blacks was to increase black hospitals and clinics, and medical and nursing schools. The Fund hoped the black medical and hospital force it was nurturing would remedy other areas it viewed as pressing for blacks, such as maternal and infant mortality.[26] Throughout the 1930s, the Fund spent the bulk of its health allotment expanding buildings and equipment of black hospitals to increase their quality and capacity to educate black physicians and trained nurses. Prior to 1930, however, it was exceedingly difficult for black physicians to gain any form of employment with public health agencies, particularly throughout the South. To throw light on the serious shortage of black public health physicians, in 1932 the Fund sponsored an American Medical Association survey of the distribution of the approximately one thousand black medical school graduates throughout the South. It also funded part of the salary of black doctors eventually added to state health departments in Texas, Louisiana, and North Carolina, as well as the municipal departments of Louisville, Baltimore, and High Point (N.C.).[27]

But the Rosenwald Fund was far more successful with its campaign among state health departments throughout the South to convince them to add black public health nurses, the expenses for which would be partially assumed by the Fund. By 1929, the Fund had approached all of the southern state health officers with this offer. Arkansas, Florida, Mississippi, Georgia, North Carolina, Tennessee, and Virginia agreed. Soon after, South Carolina, Kentucky, Louisiana, and Maryland also fell in line. By 1930 there were about forty black nurses in these state's public health operations.[28]

Although the quantitative growth in black public health nurses during the 1920s was modest, their regional and organizational spread, and impact on local public health services was substantial. In 1924 there were 365 blacks among the nation's 11,171 public health nurses. By 1931 they still numbered only 549 of the total 20,000 public health nurses.[29] But the number of cities and states employing black community nurses had spread remarkably. By 1930, the 471 black public health nurses in the North and South worked primarily for boards of health (62 and 50 percent, respectively) and public health nursing associations (36.5 and 36.4 percent). In the North a greater number of black public health nurses were employed by public schools (13) compared to the South's black nurses (7), while in the South more black nurses tended to work in tuberculosis associations.

The black public health nurse was frequently the lone black employee at the agency, but each performed a multitude of tasks and usually inspired mass community cooperation with white-controlled health care projects and clinics. Dorothy Deming, a national leader in public health nursing, gave this account of three month's activities that the typical solo black nurse completed for one county in the South:

Inspection—1,405 school children
Inspection—63 pre-school children
Home visits to 99 expectant mothers
Group conferences with 51 midwives
Typhoid immunization—84 children
Home visits to 24 cases of tuberculosis
Home visits to 10 cases of syphilis
Added to these direct services were 44 meetings of various groups, churches, lodges, etc., during which the nurse was in touch with 1,683 people.[30]

In the cities, the work responsiblity for black public health nurses was equally exhausting. For example, the black nurse responsible for community outreach at the Phipps Institute during 1920–21 conducted over 1,100 home visits in twelve months.[31] The number and range of tasks shouldered by these nurses was especially large in neighborhoods and counties not served by hospitals or permanent clinics. In the South, some of the nurses sponsored by the Rosenwald Fund had as many as eight counties under their lone supervision.[32]

During the 1920s the black public health nurse was particularly important to the nation's major urban hospitals involved in treatment and research on diseases riddling local black communities. In 1927 Landis described the extraordinary power these black women exerted at his institution, regardless of the particular medical service the facility operated. "Nearly all that is now published on this subject has dealt specifically with the tuberculosis problem and only casual mention has been made of [these nurses'] other health activities." It was the black public health nurse who also successfully encouraged black mothers to bring their children in for treatment, as well as got cooperation of teachers and pupils in local black schools to conduct examinations for infectious diseases among these children. "The educational value of these nurses is great," Landis emphasized. He found that black nurses

can arouse an interest and a desire for a knowledge of health matters among their own people that the white nurse cannot create. Just why this should be so is difficult to understand as there are many white nurses and physicians who have a keen interest and a sympathetic understanding for the negro; nevertheless it is a fact. What is of importance is the fact that where the white nurse fails the colored nurse succeeds.[33]

By the end of the decade, both black and white public health authorities praised the emergence of the black public health professional strata. On many occasions, Midian Bousfield seconded Landis's view that the medical field should broaden their employment of black public health nurses: "The greatest possible appreciation of the Negro Public Health Nurse [sic] is to be urged upon everyone. Their work to date has been largely a demonstration or an experiment which should be marked up as completely successful. There now needs to be a strong cooperative effort to extend the work so brilliantly begun."[34]

Louis Dublin also stressed repeatedly that the black doctor must be placed at the center of any efforts to reduce disease and ill-health in the black community. He expressed this message forcefully during 1928 in an overview of the health problems of blacks he wrote for *Opportunity*. Discussing the future effort to remedy the chief "health handicaps" facing black America—tuberculosis, syphilis, and high infant mortality—he placed the black physician at its center. "In the campaign which must be launched, the role of the Negro physician is supreme," Dublin wrote, "[h]e has the future of the whole race in his keeping." Although recognizing that black physicians resented the racial barriers they faced in training and practice, Dublin felt that such discrimination would remain in place for some time. "While there should be no attempt to establish racial boundaries in medical practice, it is, nevertheless, true that in sickness, the chief reliance of the colored people is upon physicians of their own people," wrote Dublin. Most important was the tremendous reverence and cultural power that black physicians had potential to garner from the black masses. "The colored physician touches the life of his race at many more points than does the average white doctor," Dublin remarked. "He speaks to them in their own terms and in a language which they clearly understand; hence his words carry greater authority and his teaching taken more seriously, I believe."[35]

During the 1920s and early 1930s, the nation's major philanthropists, the new hospital-based specialist physicians, and municipalities with the largest black communities (*not* the federal government) had provided the initiatives and revenues for these urban (and rural) black medical workers and health centers. Because of the effectiveness of this initial network of black public health professionals, a central role for black physicians and public health nurses in future community and government-sponsored health was now assured. Some cities and charities had waged effective local battles to spread health information and bring the suspected ill into appropriate medical care facilities, collect valuable cross-racial morbidity data, and spread the ideal of scientific medicine throughout substantial segments of the urban black population. But the larger epidemiological, medical, and sociological problem of excess disease mortality of blacks persisted throughout the nation. Medical authorities in federal government—through new agencies involved with disease research, public health programs, and relief measures for the massive unemployed segment—saw no choice but to step forward and try to resolve this crisis.

Part II

Federal Missions, Racial Realities

Chapter 4

The Nation-State Confronts the Black Health Crisis: Depression Through New Deal

The 1930s marked the first time a national effort to curtail the excess disease mortality among blacks emerged. Politically and philosophically, this public health movement was inspired by the national fitness patriotism enunicated by Presidents Herbert Hoover and Franklin D. Roosevelt. But it was the expanding national Public Health Service, with its campaign to eliminate venereal disease, and New Deal welfare agencies that spun and wove health studies and programs at both the federal and local levels, increasingly addressing the black–white health and mortality differential. By the decade's end, however, deficiencies in the federal agencies' antidisease campaigns unfolded. A tendency critical of the new federal public health response developed among the nation's black medical community.

Spearheaded by outspoken black doctors, and nursing and social work leaders, this community health activism challenged the priorities of and approaches taken by New Deal federal public health authorities to eliminate excess black mortality from TB, syphilis, and other health problems. The basis for this clash stemmed from the conflicting epidemic paradigms of the leadership of these two health care constituencies. The federal health agencies' highest priorities were investigating specific diseases and their prevalence; improving certain medical care services to treat victims (both extensions of traditional multifactorialism); and, finally, winning the support of the American citizenry and politicians for these goals.

Black community health activists, by contrast, forged a "relationist" paradigm, viewing the high prevalence of individual diseases in black communities as part of a social totality, a spectrum of health and social problems. In their minds the black city-dweller's health crisis was but one aspect of broad, erosive social phenomena stemming directly from impoverished living conditions, lack of adequate modern medical care resources, and mass allegiance to "unscientific" forms of folk health culture. Thus, the black medical profession's leadership agitated for the federal health agencies to address a wider range of black community health problems, expand drastically black Americans' access to medical services to equal that of whites, and improve professional opportunities for blacks in the medical fields. This conflict between paradigms governing the federal government's health mission and those of the black medical sector was a sure sign that black America's health crisis, and the competing strategies for solving it, would continue to fester into the 1940s.

1

As the shockwaves of the Depression jolted the already largely impoverished urban black communities, the health of blacks began to plummet anew in many areas. In 1920 the death rate for blacks had been 48.4 percent higher than whites; but in 1930 this gap grew to 52.8 percent.[1] The wave of TB fatalities that had swept through black America after World War I crested during the Depression. The disease was second only to heart disease as the leading cause of deaths of blacks nationally. Although the overall black mortality rate from TB declined from 448 per 100,000 in 1910 to 184 by 1930, it rose in 1931 (to 189), and a gaping racial discrepancy persisted throughout the 1930s. During the Depression years about one-fourth of TB deaths in the United States occurred among blacks. In the South, black mortality from TB, where they composed about 26 percent of the population, amounted to 53 percent of the total TB deaths in this region. Throughout urban America, blacks suffered about 28 percent of the TB deaths recorded in 42 large communities nationally. Despite their needs, treatment facilities for black tuberculars were hardly adequate. In 1934 there were 21,099 black deaths from TB in America but only 3,334 beds for black tuberculars. Throughout the 13 southern states in which three-fourths of the black population lived, 11,385 deaths from TB occurred among blacks, but only 1,666 beds were available for black patients.[2]

It is not surprising then that TB was still considered by many city medical and social workers involved with black clientele as the gravest threat to black health, despite the growing preoccupation of national public health, medical research and philanthropic authorities with venereal disease. During the summer of 1930 Charles H. Garvin, a leading black physician and health activist in Cleveland, wrote a blistering public commentary on the TB crisis, a disease he called "ubiquitous." Although he stressed that, overall, epidemic TB had declined substantially in cities where populations had developed natural immunity to the disease, urban black TB mortality continued to be heavy. In Chicago the black TB death rate was about two and one-half to three times higher than that of whites, while in Cleveland five to six times higher. Garvin maintained blacks were most frequently victimized by TB because they were undergoing "urbanization and tuberculization"; that is, acquiring natural immunization under harsh living conditions such as "long hours of hard labor, limited, often faulty diet, restriction in proper hospital and medical care, and faulty sanitation."[3]

Also around 1930 Cincinnati anti-TB organizations, concerned with the seriousness of the TB problem facing this city's blacks, helped a local public health physician organize a health survey of black male workers. The researcher's findings, presented in 1931 at the annual national conference of the American Public Health Association in Montreal, emphasized "[t]he outstanding communicable disease problem among Cincinnati negroes is tuberculosis, which led all other causes of death during 1930."[4]

The following year, another survey of black health, this time for New Jersey, was conducted by Ira De A. Reid, the noted sociologist, and J. A. Kenney, a Newark-based physician. They stated that "[i]n no field of Negro health is there a more serious problem than that of pulmonary tuberculosis." Reid and Kenney stressed that pulmonary TB still felled blacks at rates close to that of 1920. By contrast, the white death rate from TB had dropped by nearly one-half over the same decade.[5]

To the nation's black and white welfare and health care workers involved with black populations, the most shocking waste of life that TB caused throughout black communities was the increase in child victims of the disease. In 1930 education and health experts established that TB death rates for black children in grades five through nine were five times those of white students in similar grades. Black children between the ages of 10 and 14 suffered mortality rates from TB nine times greater than whites of the similar age group.[6] Industrial states and major cities with large black populations were especially aware of the extraordinary price TB was exacting throughout the black child population. In New Jersey, for instance, leading social workers wrote in 1932 that TB mortality rates in their state "show the terrific toll of this disease among Negro children and young adults." There blacks were but 5 percent of the state's total population, yet black children under 5 years of age were one-third of New Jersey's TB deaths in that age group; nearly one-half of the TB deaths within the 5–14 age-group; and 31 percent of the TB deaths among the 15–24 year olds.[7] In Cleveland 50 percent of the deaths from pulmonary TB among girls 15 and younger were black; for boys in this age group, blacks were nearly 60 percent.[8]

Debilitating childhood TB, once contracted, was exceedingly difficult to manage medically. Even the most advanced clinical researchers were baffled by the "racial" and familial factors as well as the unpredictable duration and intensity of TB infectiousness in a specific child. Hence, they could not advise health agencies with reasonable certainty about the length and conditions of supervision for individual children with TB.[9]

Besides TB, deaths among black Americans began to spike upward in several other general disease categories. The leading causes of death for black Americans in 1930 were heart disease, TB, nephritis (kidney inflammation), pneumonia, accidents, cancer, and syphilis. (See Table 2.1) Compared to the previous decade, general mortality for blacks from typhoid fever, diphtheria, malaria, nonres-piratory TB, so-called nervous diseases, and illnesses associated with pregnancy and early infancy appeared to decline. On the other hand, deaths of blacks increased from nephritis, syphilis, cancer, heart diseases, accidents, and homicides.[10]

These general trends, however, must be interpreted with cau-tion because mortality rates varied radically by region, sex, class, and the quality of local record-keeping. Moreover, during the inter-war period methods of classifying causes of mortality differed widely throughout the medical community. The range of causes and ail-ments falling under a general pathologic term was shifting rapidly as clinical medicine progressed and nonlethal chronic diseases were coming into prominence.[11] Thus, general mortality categories in use prior to World War II must now be construed cautiously as health indicators. For example, the increase in recorded deaths of blacks attributed to nephritis or "nephrotic syndrome" signified more than simply greater prevalence of this condition. This pattern most likely hid the prevalence of many other long-term diseases such as differ-ent forms of lupus, malaria, syphilis, hypertension, sickle cell ane-mia, or exposure to toxic materials: all of which can cause fatal kid-ney disease as an end-effect.[12]

But local public health and medical studies on black popula-tions of specific cities, states, and regions, were built on more reli-able mortality and morbidity health reportage for specific subpopulations: data on morbidity among patients seeking treatment at local hospitals, clinics, and maternity and infant care centers; and surveys completed by local public health departments with the support of the United States Public Health Service or the Julius Rosenwald Fund.[13] Local health data revealed the gap between black and white rates of contracting many serious infectious diseases had widened during the Depression years.

Infant mortality struck blacks at staggering levels even though overall rates nationwide were dropping. During the early 1930s about 250,000 black infants were born yearly, of which approximately 22,000 died each year. Over half of the black infants who died during their first year of life did so within thirty days from their birth. Authorities grouped (in rank order) the four leading causes of black infant deaths as "natal or prenatal" causes (premature births, congenital debility, injury at birth, and syphilis), respiratory diseases, gastrointestinal diseases, and communicable diseases. Geographically, from 1933 to 1935 in Oklahoma, Delaware, Kentucky, Maryland, and the District of Columbia, the average infant mortality rate for blacks exceeded 100 per 1,000 live births; it was from 90 to 99 in Missouri, Tennessee, South Carolina, Virginia, North Carolina, Florida, and Kansas; from 80 to 89 in Indiana, New York, Louisiana, Georgia, Pennsylvania, Massachusetts, Ohio, New Jersey, West Virginia, Alabama, and Texas; and slightly below 80 in Illinois, Connecticut, Mississippi, Michigan, California, and Arkansas.[14]

A widespread notion among many concerned with black health during the 1930s was that blacks from World War I through the Depression had divided primarily into a southern rural component and a northern urban component, with the rural black folk suffering the greater excess of preventable infant deaths. But actually, black infant mortality was more common in urban areas of both regions than rural ones. During the early and mid-1930s, nearly two-thirds of the nation's black infants were born in the South. A considerable number of these infant births, however, occurred in the large southern cities where child-health services were generally more sparse than in the cities of the North.[15]

The higher infant death rates experienced by blacks translated into shorter longevity for this minority as well. Louis Dublin drew on data collected between 1912 and the mid-1930s on about 2,000,000 black policyholders with Metropolitan Life. He estimated that during 1929–31 life expectancy at birth was 47.5 years for black males and 49.5 for black females, compared to 59.3 and 62.8 for whites, respectively. Dublin attributed this racial differential largely to the higher black infant mortality. "The death of a colored infant cuts off, at one stroke, 48 years of life," he stated in 1937, "and when there is a heavy infant mortality, the life expectancy is very seriously affected."[16]

In addition to high infant death rates, many blacks were dying in adulthood because of preventable conditions or communicable disease related to childbirth. Throughout the South, the mortality rate for blacks over 30 years of age actually increased from 1920 to 1930.[17] Maternal mortality struck down black women at shocking rates. Between 1933 and 1935 about 2,400 black women died each year from conditions related to pregnancy and childbirth. During 1933 and 1934 maternal death was second only to TB as the nation's leading killer of black women of general child-bearing ages (that is, 15 to 44). Elizabeth Tandy, a researcher for the Children's Bureau and a leading expert on this subject, stressed in 1937 that many black women who survive pregnancies "do so with lowered health status." Not only did black new mothers suffer more impaired health than whites, but because of blacks' generally lower economic status, the mothers' impaired health tended to affect more negatively the health of their children. "The Negro mother, even more commonly than the white mother," Tandy stated, "serves as nurse [and] an important contributor to the family income. The health and welfare of the child are recognized as wrapped in the health and well-being of the mother. This is even more true for the Negro child than for the white child."[18]

An untold range of ill-health and symptomatic patterns among black Americans during the Depression decade was going unrecorded because these ailments were caused largely by underlying economic/workplace factors. At this time, these health problems usually were not monitored by employers or public health officials. Generally, neither mortality nor morbidity data were designed to reflect the profusion of illnesses, injuries, and disabling conditions levied on the blacks in the process of laboring within the nation's chaotic industrial sector and stagnant agriculture. It is now well documented in current epidemiolgy and toxicology that both protracted exposure to unhealthy work environments (especially in manual workfields) as well as conditions of chronic unemployment destroy organs, limbs, and minds.[19] Yet it was only some years into the Depression that local and federal health authorities systematically enumerated health data in correlation with income or employment status, providing a basis for comparing urban black and white American populations.[20]

In the spring of 1933, the Milbank Memorial Fund, the Public

Health Service, and the Emergency Work and Relief Bureau of New York City assembled data on about 7,400 families in eight poor sections of major cities, as well as 2,300 black and white low-income families in New York City. This was one of the first surveys involving federal agencies on disabling illness rates for urban white and black wage-earning families.[21] The key finding was that respiratory and digestive diseases, as well as accidents were the most frequent cause of disabling illness. These rates for black New York City residents exceeded those of whites in New York City and the other six cities. Although communicable diseases were lower among the blacks surveyed, this was explained by the alleged tendency of blacks to succumb to these diseases earlier in youth, as well as a measles outbreak that had hit the white sample-group population. The surveyors stressed that overall their studies demonstrated "the sensitiveness of illness rates to slight changes in income and employment status, even when all data are confined to neighborhoods which would be judged as 'poor' by present-day standards."[22]

Many public health authorities and major insurance companies considered the syphilis case and mortality rates for black Americans cause for alarm. In 1934 syphilis was blamed for causing about 17,700 deaths. Also, there were an estimated 7,000,000 persons with syphilis, meaning that about one of every ten adults would have the disease during his or her life. About 500,000 new cases were entering treatment annually. Louis Dublin called syphilis a "major public health problem in the United States [whose] ravages . . . are greatest among colored persons." He estimated that the syphilis death rate for black males was approximately four times greater than for white; for black females, about six times greater than for white. In urban areas, the black-to-white ratio for syphilis was reported as high as ten to one.[23]

2

Although in the early 1930s the black–white mortality differential from TB and syphilis was widening, federal agencies, major philanthropies, and many cities were finally open to at least debate the black American's health predicament. Some of these segments even began measures to assess more accurately the source for this discrepancy, and or expand preventive and curative treatment.

Among the first federal bodies to discuss publicly the high levels of communicable disease throughout urban rural black communities was President Hoover's White House Conference on Child

Health and Protection. This gathering was organized in November 1930 because of Hoover's strong political philosophy that healthy children were the vital root for a democratic nation. Believing that the federal government should exercise only minimal control over America's business and civic affairs, President Hoover's national health ethos stressed popular hygiene and a fit workforce. At the opening of the conference, Hoover gave one of the most noteworthy speeches of his career. It centered on the importance of safeguarding America's children. "[H]ealthier minds in more vigorous bodies," Hoover exclaimed, were necessary "to direct the energies of our Nation to yet greater heights of achievement." Improved national health, beginning with fit children, would also lessen the shackles of government growth. "If we could have but one generation of properly born, trained, educated, and healthy children, a thousand other problems of government would vanish. . . . Moreover, one good community nurse will save a dozen future policemen."[24]

The administrative official most supportive of placing black health problems on the White House Conference agenda, as well as inviting black social welfare professionals to the affair, was Secretary of the Interior Ray Lyman Wilbur. A renowned university administrator, medical doctor, public policy adviser for the medical profession, and Hoover confidant, Wilbur believed pragmatically that federal health programs could not ignore the black's health problems.[25] His department had continuous direct involvement with black health affairs because it administered both the Freedmen's Hospital and Howard University, which had America's leading black medical college. Throughout his tenure heading the Department of the Interior, Wilbur supported expanding these institutions as well as other health education projects throughout the nation's black communities.[26]

Although the conference's 1,100 participants were divided under three major sections (medical service, public health service, and education and training), black community workers were employed both as members of sessions and outside advisers to the conference only in the last category. Nonetheless, compared to Theodore Roosevelt's White House conference in 1909 and Woodrow Wilson's in 1919, Hoover's was, according to Wilbur, "the first which may acknowledge the positive cooperation and participation of Negro experts in child care." Wilbur reasoned that black welfare professionals had an enormous task on their hands in nourishing fit and well-adjusted black children, and that their involvement in the conference was a benefit "to the colored people and of great importance to the country as a whole."[27]

Despite the limited role allocated to black welfare experts —apparently no black physicians were invited as major participants—they and the white conference leaders brought the health issue to the fore of the meeting's concerns.[28] In their general statement, the conveners made specific references to the critical health and social needs of America's blacks: "The whole problem of Negro health is still a difficult one to solve, and much study is being given to it by many groups." The conference leaders underscored the national extent of this issue: "It is to be hoped definite information may be secured, for it must be remembered that the health of the Negro population . . . concerns nearly 10 percent of our total population, and the health of the Negro has a direct influence on the general health of the community."[29]

The conference leaders reviewed a study and report prepared in the planning phase of the conference on the efficacy of black hospitals and medical personnel to address the health needs of the nation's black population. While most of these hospitals were located in the South where the majority of American blacks were still concentrated, the convenors found "they are largely given over to surgical cases." "There is little provision for [general] medical cases or children," the report emphasized. Only 24 (or 13 percent) of the 183 such institutions were fully accredited.[30] Measured against the nation's overall hospital resources of about 6,665 approved hospitals supplying well over one million beds, the 9,027 beds provided by these black hospitals were a miniscule weapon against mass disease throughout typical black American communities.[31] The conferees recommended as more practical increasing the number of black public health nurses along the lines of the Phipps Institute's successful approaches in this area.[32]

When Eugene Kinckle Jones, executive secretary of the National Urban League addressed one of the sessions on "Special Child Groups," he drew from the long experience the League had in monitoring and publicizing inadequate health conditions of city blacks. He believed that three developments were causing the high numbers of dependent black children throughout urban America. First, the Great Migration drawing blacks into the cities had overburdened the welfare resources of these municipalities. Second, in the major cities, "the constitution of the Negro family" tended to produce a large population of children lacking the benefits of close parental supervision. Because of economic necessity, black women worked almost twice as frequently as their white counterparts. Moreover, since rates of illegitimate births were especially high among blacks, there are

"20,000 Negro children born each year of unmarried mothers, and the [poor] economic background, we feel, is largely responsible for this."[33]

Finally, Jones emphasized that housing resources were particularly inadequate for urban blacks and new immigrants. Several unhealthy conditions prevailed in the housing of city blacks: buildings tended to be aging and in disrepair; dwellings lacked "sanitary provisions"; subdivision of houses was common, creating too many tenants or the "lodger evil"; and the neighborhoods of blacks typically did not receive "street cleaning and street paving, garbage disposal and lighting, and so forth."[34]

Eugene Jones and the other black civic activists at the White House Conference called for expanding assistance to black mothers and children to ameliorate the impact of these unwholesome social conditions, as well as expanding the use of newly trained black social work personnel to improve black community children services. Jones also entreated all social welfare organizations in black neighborhoods or with substantial black clientele to have "mixed boards of control" and "Negro representation in administration and support of these agencies." Another forceful voice was that of Sally Stewart, the president of the National Association of Colored Women.[35] She also stressed building cohesiveness within the black family as the optimal means for rehabilitating the immediate environment surrounding impoverished children. Calling attention to her thirty-four years of social work with black children, Stewart emphasized that upgrading the lives of these children had to be "built in the Negro home, and [with] intelligent motherhood [to] protect the child in the primitive and formative years of his life."[36]

The White House Conference had raised expectations that black health and social welfare concerns would receive broad support, at least from the executive branch. But only a few months after the meeting, as Hoover's public support slid precipitously among Americans hurt by the economic crash, black community workers criticized it as an exercise in futility since the federal government did not follow up concretely on conference recommendations. Nonetheless, Urban League officials held that the conference represented some accomplishment. "This was the first conference which has given any considerable attention to the most handicapped child in America," League officials wrote, "[a]nd that in itself is no little progress."[37]

The White House Conference and the Rosenwald Fund projects described earlier had begun to edge the black health crisis onto the federal agenda of public health issues. However, federal agencies that would conduct New Deal projects addressing black community health problems had not yet formed. Still, following the trends of the 1920s, various efforts to stem the TB scourge among urban blacks continued to emerge from municipal health centers and districts, usually combining with black community-based lay health initiatives or medical institutions. By 1930 there were some 1,511 health centers operating throughout the nation. The majority had been established during the 1910s and 1920s, financed by public revenues and, to a lesser extent, community chests, philanthropic funds, or voluntary donations. Most (729) were directed by municipal or county departments of health, or nonprofit agencies (725). Sporadically the municipal health centers and districts confronted with large black populations collected information on the mass disease problems of this group, occasionally providing a patchwork of limited services for blacks.[38]

In Baltimore, for example, during 1932 and 1933 the director of the city health department's tuberculosis bureau, B. T. Baggott, assessed data on the TB problems of black Baltimore residents, concluding the situation was "still very serious." Although blacks were 18 percent of the city's population, they represented over 50 percent of the TB deaths in Baltimore. The Tuberculosis Dispensary was Baltimore's central examination and treatment facility for persons suspected of having clinical TB. In 1932 and again in 1933 this center treated about 1,450 new patients referred by private physicians, city agencies, and charitable organizations. But although blacks did receive examinations for TB, long-term treatment facilities and sanitorium beds for blacks both locally and statewide were virtually nonexistent.[39]

Furthermore, Baltimore health officials were fatalistic about the possibility of finding any clear solutions for lowering the TB menace in the city's black sections. Blacks "are essentially a home loving race, and reluctantly remain in an institution when sent there," Baggott stated. "On the other hand, there are insufficient beds for their accommodation, particularly for Negro children, and it is among the children where the most good can be accomplished. The natural and environmental factors of tuberculosis among adult Negroes robs them of their chance for ultimate recovery."[40]

Blacks in Depression-era New York City were relatively more fortunate in obtaining TB screening and treatment resources compared to other cities. Public health authorities there frequently united with philanthropic organizations to publicize the seriousness of the

TB problem in the city's black communities, and took definite measures to curtail this threat. TB deaths in the city had climbed from 1927 to 1933, and the mortality rate for blacks from the disease was over double the white rate. Manhattan, although with only one-fourth of the city's total population, had nearly one-half of New York City's TB deaths in 1933. From 1929 to 1931 about 5,000 new cases of pulmonary TB were reported yearly in Manhattan. Within this large TB problem, black New York was faring even worse. According to one study sponsored by the Phelps–Stokes Fund, the 1929–31 TB mortality data for Manhattan revealed that "[m]ost, but not all of the areas with high tuberculosis death rates, had a large colored population with extremely high tuberculosis rates."[41]

Treatment facilities for TB victims in Manhattan were substantial although frequently overtaxed, and Harlem blacks helped establish a systematic channel to information about (and often admission to) these services. There were eleven TB clinics in Manhattan, publicly and privately financed; twenty hospitals and sanitoriums in New York City or nearby giving free or low-cost TB care to the city's residents; and one of the nation's most active private anti-TB organizations, the New York Tuberculosis and Health Association.[42]

As mentioned earlier, shortly after World War I the Tuberculosis Association had combined with local black medical professionals and established the Harlem Tuberculosis and Health Committee. Initially headquartered in the Urban League building in Harlem, the Health Committee's TB component served primarily as an information and referral service to assist neighborhood physicians in placing patients in sanitoriums. They referred about 1,000 persons each year to appropriate medical facilities and disseminated public health information throughout the community. The Health committee also followed the Phipps Institute example and employed a public health nurse (trained at the Institute) who conducted community outreach services.[43]

Similar to earlier black community-based centers originally established to combat either TB or venereal disease, the Health Committee gradually expanded into a multipurpose, albeit unofficial public health center. Such centers were highly visible in the health affairs of its surrounding black community. But these centers were also politically impotent, as they were disconnected from the staffing and policy-making power as well as from government revenues controlled within the municipal public health system. By 1930, the Health Committee had added other operations, including a dental clinic and postgraduate "institutes" for local general physicians on

TB, venereal diseases, and heart diseases. These institutes were a means for neighborhood doctors, generally barred by race from specialty training in medical schools, to update their technical skills in the diagnosis and treatment of these diseases. One New York Tuberculosis Association official described a typical institute as "lectures and observation classes, open to the physicians of Harlem, which are held in the various hospitals and clinics" conducted by specialists. Furthermore, the Health Committee had broadened its educational campaigns to social clubs, industrial sites, and youth and parental groups. By the mid-1930s the Health Committee was viewed as "practically a public health agency."[44]

Unlike Baltimore, which lacked both a fully organized TB bureau and a system of facilities large enough to service its heavily populated black communities, or Philadelphia, which relied primarily on a small network of special TB clinics for blacks operated charitably by the Phipps Institute, Cleveland had developed one of the most comprehensive public TB control programs in the nation.[45] Yet, as described in Chapter 3, the Cleveland system lacked a special program to reach blacks who likely had infectious (clinical) TB.

Indeed, the Cleveland program epitomized the limits of rigid or hyperbolic multifactorialism. Even with its umbrella of TB examination and treatment services, managing city residents known to be tuberculous proved a task of immense complexity. The Cleveland TB program included a comprehensive, intricately layered system of files serving as a registry of all cases, their stage of sickness, and information on follow-up contacts. One set of case records for patients was kept at the district TB clinic that treated these individuals, and a copy also maintained in the central city health office. The central municipal files also included case records on all cases under treatment at privately operated health services, thereby ensuring a comprehensive information system for surveillance and planning purposes. Health workers, medical specialists, and nurses collectively applied the environmentalist approach, striving to trace and "seal" infectious agents within individual carriers throughout the city's multitudes. Each cell within the public health system functioned to administer to one of the factors: the physician identified the clinically infected individual; nurses and clerks followed the patient's compliance with treatments; the social case worker counseled the families of the tubercular to minimize interaction with their infectious relative; and administrative personnel of the city health department assured overall efficient availability of services and careful cross-institutional surveillance of treatment records.[46]

But Cleveland's TB program lacked substantial black medical and counseling personnel, a precondition for attracting blacks suspected of having TB into its complicated pipeline of diagnostic and treatment services. Not surprisingly this city continued to have one of the nation's most extreme black–white TB mortality ratios (about five or six to one) during the early 1930s. Local TB authorities attributed the city's slow overall drop in TB mortality to the high frequency of deaths due to the disease among its growing black population.[47] The Cleveland program, then, represented the most advanced (potentially) as well as less effective (actually) municipal initiatives against the TB scourge afflicting urban blacks.

Throughout the South, TB treatment facilities and sanitoriums for blacks were grossly inadequate, segregated by law as well as institutional practice, and considered by black and white medical authorities involved in black health affairs a national disaster. Although in this region the black mortality rate from TB was about four times greater compared to whites, blacks had only one-fifth the hospital beds than whites had for TB care.[48] In 1936 the National Tuberculosis Association published the results of its five-year study of TB among blacks. It revealed that in some southern states the ratio of black deaths from TB to available hospital beds for TB patients was as high as twenty to one. Clarence H. Payne, a leading Chicago black physician involved in the TB issue, wrote a letter to Claude A. Barnett, the head of the Associated Negro Press, seeking wider national support for black fund-raising efforts to counter this "stark tragedy in the Southland."[49]

3

Local efforts to curtail epidemic diseases among urban blacks varied in quality, depending mostly on "bottom up" factors such as the presence of strong-willed community health activists or a municipality's capacity to recognize and address the health needs of its black poor. By contrast, the national medical establishment's response to the high TB and syphilis rates among black Americans was controlled from the "top down" by two forces: the governing epidemic paradigm and (often implicit) sociological theories followed by the health–sciences research community; and the politics, priorities, and organizational forms within the federal health and welfare agencies that actualized these paradigms. During the Depression and New Deal both American medicine and federal health officials fixed even more firmly on multifactorial paradigms.

Even throughout this period of economic and social collapse, many health authorities believed as strongly as ever that infectious-disease patterns were beating clearly distinct paths in the urban populations because of "racial factors." Virtually all medical authorities admitted that the material deprivation attending the Depression had a broad negative effect on the health of unemployed Americans. But most clinical researchers, biologists, and social scientists still held that both susceptibility to and effects of TB and syphilis were to a strong degree racially determined. Indeed, as this section will show, the most popular paradigm of public health authorities of the 1930s and early 1940s, Parran's seroepidemiology, was merely a static amalgam of the two multifactorial idea-systems: anatomic-genetics and environmentalism.

Throughout the 1930s Eugene Opie and his followers continued to stress anatomic, constitutional factors as determinative in the black–white TB mortality differential. While Opie agreed that poverty and TB were closely associated, he still emphasized the racial-physiological dimension of the TB problem. As late as 1936, he and two coresearchers described what they believed were significant racial differences in clinical TB cases they encountered. "Are the numerical relations between clinically manifest TB . . . attending our clinic applicable to the general population?" they queried. They believed yes, arguing that one could expect similar differences to run throughout the larger populations with "the intellectual, economic and racial constitution of the families under the care of the [Phipps Institute] dispensary."[50]

The anatomical research on TB in racial groups by Opie and his Phipps coworkers was complemented during the 1930s by the studies of Everett, and Pinner and Kasper, many of which were published in the *American Review of Tuberculosis*.[51] In 1932 the latter two researchers, for instance, studied postmortem reports of black patients in Detroit and Chicago presumed to have died from TB. They were most impressed by the high rate in which lymphatic tissues were involved as well as the frequency of acute and severe exudative reactions to the tubercle bacilli infection. The Pinner–Kasper study pointed out that while this reaction (they termed it hematogenous dissemination) also occured in whites, it was far less frequent: "[T]o produce a composite picture of what TB does in the Negro and in the whites, it would have to be said that one extreme is presented by strictly localized fibrotic lesion, 'isolated phthisis,' and the other by massive exudative lesions and by hematogenous and lymphogenous spread."[52]

Another body of 1930s medical research that continued to emphasize anatomic, and implicitly, immutable genetic distinctions between blacks and whites grew in and around the work of Raymond Pearl. Through the mid-1930s Pearl remained one of the nation's most long-standing and influential minds committed to phrenology. He was an anatomist who favored zealously establishing "biometric constants" that distinguish the size and weight of brains of blacks and whites. "It is an accepted view," he stated in 1934, "that the skull capacity and the brain weight of the Negro, whether pure or mixed with white races, tends on the average to be smaller than the same dimensions in whites."[53]

Believing they were combining medical analysis and physical anthropology, Pearl and other anatomists laboriously collected data to verify cranial and other anatomic capacities that differentiated the black American (African) and white races. Moreover, Pearl still relied heavily on the earlier studies by the controversial physician-researcher Robert B. Bean, a forefather of American craniometrics; as well as on F. W. Vint's research on the skull capacity of several hundred Kenyan adults.[54] Pearl contended race traits superseded national origins or centuries-old intermingling of peoples; and argued for a step-up in the gathering of "quantitative material on variation in man, in respect of various anatomical and physiological characteristics."[55] The differences Pearl alleged he found in brain size for blacks in comparison to whites were more fundamental than those thus far uncovered for other body organs: the "liver, kidneys, spleen, heart, appendix or pancreas." He thus urged that, except for newly emerging genetics, phrenological study of blacks was the most promising field in anatomical quantification and classification of races. "The smoothness of the figures" that established smaller brain weights for blacks, Pearl wrote in *Science* magazine, "has enticed me into struggling to rationalize them genetically, but I have had no success. . . . Perhaps some ingenious reader can do better."[56]

Influential American sociologists and human biologists through the mid-1930s also continued to mine the hereditarian field, providing theoretical hyperbole and social data complementary to medicine's racial anatomy. Samuel Holmes strengthened his earlier racialist theories explaining black–white TB mortality. In a 1937 study of the leading causes of mortality among blacks, Holmes, citing the work of Pearl, Smillie and Augustine, and others, emphasized that black Americans apparently possessed lungs with "distinctly less" capacity than those of whites. "How far the Negro's so-called 'tropical lung' may predispose him to tuberculosis is uncertain," he submitted.[57] Indeed, general mortality data indicated clear declines in TB mortality for both whites and blacks. Furthermore, environmentalist explanations for disease mortality were gaining increasing credibility in medical and sociological circles. Holmes acknowledged there was significant uncertainty in medical and biological research about the specific causes for the higher rate of black TB deaths. He also conceded that black TB mortality had declined substantially in recent years. But he merely dug deeper into racialist conceptualizations, contending that genotypical racial distinctions ultimately determined the superior health of whites, that genetic inheritance not only controlled constitution but human immunity as well.

To explain high TB mortality of blacks, Holmes and other social biologists now simply controlled for the broadest environmental variables, say, rural/urban residence or income level.[58] They then shifted their analysis to emphasize racial constitution as the remaining key determinant of TB mortality and, if necessary, other types of mortality (lobar pneumonia especially) in which the racial disparity had seemed to widen. On the one hand, Holmes recognized that "[t]he matter of racial susceptibility is, of course, complicated by the fact that the unfavorable status of the Negro has the effect of enhancing the death rate from respiratory infections, as from most other diseases." But instead of using only the hereditarian concept to explain why members of the black "race" had weaker physical endowments compared to whites, he now accented three chief elements. Note his rather circumspect opening: "Under present conditions there are two, and not improbably three, important factors involved in the differential mortality of Negroes and whites from respiratory diseases: (1) external factors, such as food, climate, care, etc.; (2) previous immunization due to contact with infective germs; and (3) racial heredity."[59]

In his major work, *The Negro's Struggle For Survival* (1937), Holmes placed greatest emphasis on the "selective action of disease," particularly TB, pneumonia, and venereal disease. These ailments struck blacks most frequently, Holmes maintained, because genetically they were less immune than whites. Making broad deductions from animal biology, Holmes claimed there were no "human made" factors that could ultimately outweigh racial susceptibility. He recognized minimal infections could yield natural immunities that protected large populations from TB. But Holmes still stressed that "the important role of genetic factors in disease resistance, which has been demonstrated in different races of plants and animals, makes it very likely *a priori* that races so different as the Negro and the Caucasian may differ in their reactions to [TB's] pathogenic agencies."[60] During the 1930s, major researchers of infectious diseases and race considered Holmes's work irrefutable sociological and biological validation of race distinctions.[61]

Despite the enduring strength of medical and sociological racialism, the less-popular environmentalist paradigm continued to gain support throughout the Depression decade. This was especially true of the public and medical communities responding to the high level of black TB mortality. Increasingly, environmental epidemiology and social welfare studies superseded or leveled discursive blows directly against the phenotypical or anatomic-genetic explanations for higher black TB deaths as argued by Pearl.

The boldest assaults on racialist epidemiology of TB were by the still-growing cluster of white and black specialists. Situated mostly at large urban hospitals, they were able to study morbidity patterns derived from their own hospital experiences and racially and socially diverse patient populations. Vital statistics amassed by local and federal government units on long-term demographic patterns were increasingly accurate. In prior decades such data had been sparse, due largely to the undeveloped state of hospital morbidity records and federal census reporting, and also to the lack of a federal system for registering morbidity. Yet it is precisely information on milder, subclinical prevalence, and untreated cases that tends to close confounding gaps in explaining differing patterns in the spread of and mortality from epidemic diseases.[62]

During the Depression years a growing number of physician-researchers involved in TB clinics for blacks questioned seriously why so many in medicine continued to focus on establishing racial or constitutional factors for the higher black TB mortality. Charles Garvin criticized those medical and social work authorities who were predicting that because the industrial depression had thrown thousands of black workers out of jobs and sanitary environments, America's black race would inevitably decline. He called these pessimists "overzealous health propagandists." While Garvin was concerned about the current high levels of TB among city blacks, he reaffirmed that blacks were collectively surviving. He deemed Frederick Hoffman the "Prophet of Negro Extinction" whom "[t]ime has proven . . . to be in error." To Garvin, popular arguments about "predisposition, that constitutional anomaly, the possessor of which succumbs readily in the struggle with infectious germs," were only "cowardly modes of escaping from the consideration of the effect of physical and social influences upon the human races."[63]

Moreover, as early as 1931 no clear evidence existed verifying greater or less susceptiblity to TB in individuals belonging to certain blood groups. As Julian H. Lewis, the outstanding pathologist of Provident Hospital (Chicago) stated, "the blood-group index of Negroes is unrelated to their reaction to TB."[64] Meanwhile, other physician-researchers and social workers had continued to produce microstudies indicating the pivotal influence of housing congestion and poverty on the spread of TB. In 1932 the noted black sociologist Ira De A. Reid codirected a statewide survey of TB among blacks in New Jersey. He and coresearcher Beatrice A. Myers called for a new public dialogue and policy approach to the TB epidemic, stressing improved social and health conditions for blacks. "It is becoming more and more apparent as research advances that TB is a disease of poverty and ignorance," they wrote, "[y]et when the question of TB among Negroes is discussed, it is too often taken for granted that the high death rate in this group is due not to environmental factors but to some 'racial susceptibility.'"[65]

Medical and public health authorities were no longer surprised to find TB death rates high in slum neighborhoods because the disease seemed fanned particularly by impoverished living situations. During the mid-1930s George G. Ornstein, a physician at New York Post Graduate Medical School of Columbia University and adviser to the city on TB facilities for local blacks, researched TB among blacks of specific occupational groups.[66] His findings helped devastate the widely held racialist idea that blacks suffered more frequently from an acute and rapidly fatal type of TB.[67] Writing in a special issue on black health in Howard University's *Journal of Negro Education* (1937), Ornstein called "'racial susceptibility'" and "'racial resistance' . . . vague terms . . . that up to the present no investigators have been able to explain . . . with clarity in relation to TB infection in the Negro race compared to the white race."[68]

Ornstein cited the great reduction in TB rates among Irish immigrants to New York City—who as early as 1920 suffered TB death rates of 306 per 100,000—once they began to move out of over-crowded living conditions and poverty. He urged the medical community to direct greatest attention to the environmental factors conducive to TB infection: "We know the improvement which took place in the slum sections of the white race in all large cities, and we should be hopeful for similar results when both the economic and environmental conditions of the Negro are changed for the better."[69]

A few years later the Phelps–Stokes Fund coordinated and published a massive, exacting study of New York City housing and health. Stressing what it termed architectual conditions and activities

within the home, the study established the strong association
between crowded, ill-heated, poorly lit housing, and the high levels
of TB mortality occurring in neighborhoods of poor blacks and
newly arriving Puerto Rican immigrants. Housing had "an important
bearing either upon the acquisition of certain diseases or upon
recovery from them." Breaking from the conventional focus of medical authorities on infectious disease as the central public health
problem, the study analyzed disease patterns under five groups: (1)
"traumatic," which included injuries and lesions; (2) "chemical toxic,"
pertaining to, for instance, carbon monoxide poisoning; (3) "parasitic," such as hookworm, tapeworm, malaria, yellow fever; (4) "bacterial" (and viral), including conjunctivitis (transmitted, for example,
by roller-towels) and respiratory ailments such as TB; and (5) "nervous" disorders, such as "mental upset" due to fear of house fires,
and eye and ear strain due to poor lighting or noise pollution. The
Phelps–Stokes report emphasized that while housing conditions
were the primary cause of such diseases, they were never the sole
cause. It acknowleged some influence of "constitutional predisposition, hereditary or acquired," but cautioned that "[e]ach illness is a
resultant of the interplay of many factors operating within the individual and within his physical and social environment."[70]

While public health newcomers increasingly argued that the
greater TB deaths of blacks derived from environment, they were
much less certain about the role of race in another epidemic that
also appeared to single out America's blacks: venereal diseases. During the early 1930s, morbidity data from hospitals, physicians (particularly those with obstetrical practices), major insurance companies,
and the Rosenwald Fund–Public Health Service demonstrations and
surveys pointed to syphilis as the leading public health crisis facing
blacks and the nation.[71] In 1933, Baltimore municipal health officials,
for example, were more dismayed about the city's inability to control venereal disease among its black residents than the local TB crisis. That year city health authorities studied the local incidence of
and mortality from TB and syphilis since 1924. They found syphilis
cases greatly exceeded TB ones, and that mortality caused by the
two diseases were approaching the same level (see Figure 4.1). During 1924 to 1933 the ratio of syphilis mortality for blacks to whites
was on average ten to one, compared to TB mortality of only three
to one. As for incidence rates of venereal disease, that is, cases per
100,000 population, syphilis among blacks was nine times higher
than whites; chancroid, seventeen times higher for blacks; and gonorrhea, four times higher.[72]

FIGURE 4.1

Cases and Deaths from Syphilis and Tuberculosis in
the Black Population of Baltimore, 1924–1933

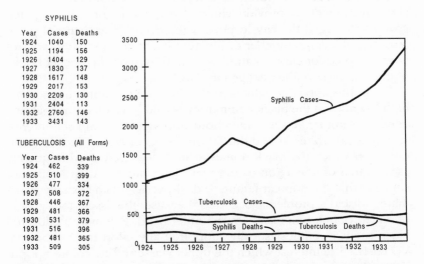

SYPHILIS

Year	Cases	Deaths
1924	1040	150
1925	1194	156
1926	1404	129
1927	1830	137
1928	1617	148
1929	2017	153
1930	2209	130
1931	2404	113
1932	2760	146
1933	3431	143

TUBERCULOSIS (All Forms)

Year	Cases	Deaths
1924	462	339
1925	510	399
1926	477	334
1927	508	372
1928	446	367
1929	481	366
1930	531	379
1931	516	396
1932	481	365
1933	509	305

Source: F. O. Reinhard, "Bureau of Venereal Disease," *City of Baltimore, One Hundred and Nineteenth Annual Report of the Health Department —1933*, 98.

The director of the Baltimore health department's bureau of venereal disease, Ferdinand O. Reinhard, summarized the grim situation facing the black community in 1933. The black residential districts in Baltimore were concentrated in the western and eastern sides of the city. The western district, Reinhard said, has "the characteristics of a self-contained city and can be readily compared to the Harlem section of New York." Like the white population, both black communities had a three-class structure: an "intelligentsia" relatively smaller than that of the white community; "a fair sized middle class"; and largest of all, a "proleterian [class] . . . engaged in laboring work." It was this latter segment that was experiencing the brunt of the venereal disease devastation. "This group has suffered severely under the depression," Reinhard stated, "and is actually existing near the bread line."[73]

Baltimore health officials responsible for venereal disease and TB services implored the larger white community to try to understand the practical implications presented by the venereal disease and TB epidemic among the city's black residents. Since venereal diseases eventually resulted in victims seriously impaired by heart disease, insanity, and neurological disorders, the economic impact of these diseases was severe. In his 1933 ten-year review of Baltimore's black community and the venereal disease problem, Reinhard emphasized that "[f]or purely selfish reasons, it would be wise for a city government to provide clinics for the care of this forgotten group." He urged the city to ponder the even larger financial problems that this large number of indigent black patients "who are not now accepted for clinic treatment [would] have on the pocket books of the taxpayers of the next generation."[74]

But this appeal to whites to consider the economic impact that high VD rates in the black community would have on municipal revenues did not strike the same chord of pragmatism and self-interest among local whites as had the TB outbreaks of earlier decades, outbreaks in which the black domestic strata was perceived frequently as a source of contagion to the white community. Allan M. Brandt suggests that the popular failure to deal publicly with sexually transmitted disease problems occurred because the issue too greatly offended popular morals.[75] On the other hand, Baltimore's educated black segment enthusiastically supported any effort to confront the VD crisis. "The interest which the upper classes of the colored population show in the problems which affect the welfare of their race, and the cooperation shown towards any effort made to help them solve their own problem," noted Reinhard, "is one of the most heartening aspects of this [the local VD control] picture."[76] Tapping this interest, in 1934 the Baltimore health department initiated a sex education program targeted for the city's blacks. It included exhibits for Negro Health Week and the National Association of Teachers in Colored Schools, presentations at local black high schools, and distribution of thousands of pamphlets.[77]

Reinhard also stressed the benefits of using black medical professionals: "Experience based on a period of ten years, has shown that in Baltimore colored patients prefer to be treated by colored physicians." The reason for this was in substance cultural, although Reinhard cast it in racial terms. "This is unquestionably due to a psychological understanding of racial problems which the average white physician does not possess." The same type of rapport became evident in the area of nursing services and social casework.[78] Reinhard compared the track records of black and white caseworkers doing so-called social investigation:

For example, one colored social investigator working with colored women, has been able in a period of six months to ferret

out 56 contacts of 50 cases. Of these, 38 showed evidence of
syphilis and are now under treatment. Seven of the remaining
were positive for gonorrhea. So far, no white social worker has
been able to get results remotely comparable.[79]

By the close of 1934, however, public health authorities of both
urban and rural communities found the prevalence of syphilis so
widespread, they viewed it as economically impossible to provide
comprehensive screening and treatment programs.[80] The stage was
set for the federal health agencies to take the lead in fighting the
syphilis threat as well as other health problems of the nation's working masses. But there could be neither medical scientific, nor public
health progress among the black American ill without the means to
interconnect with this national minority subculture.

4

The federal government's struggle against syphilis during the
1930s was an uphill battle against conventional, middle-class social
and sexual values which were resistant to recognizing the biomedical nature of venereal diseases. But this struggle against conservative
social morals was only one theater in the national health agencies'
war against venereal disease. A more essential theater, federal health
authorites believed, was the syphilis epidemic running amock
throughout black American populations. To these health leaders a
triumph on the racial front—that is, explaining why and how the
syphilis spirochete prefered to attack a particular "racial species"
—promised great leaps in the biomedical control of syphilis. Not
only could it lead to improvements in the therapeutic power of
American medicine generally; in the long run it could sway more
politicians, employers, and social welfare workers involved with
large black populations to support the federal anti-VD initiatives.[81]
Despite the growing strength of environmentalism during the
New Deal era, the governing idea for the federal health agencies'
policy to reduce syphilis throughout the black communities
remained grounded in anatomic-genetic racialism. There were several factors conducive to the reformulation of racialism. First, traditional racialism did not pass from the intellectual scientific scene during
the interwar decades. Instead, it conveniently meshed with segrega-
tionist cultural thought and sociolegal mechanisms (what Gunnar
Myrdal termed the *anti-amalgamation doctrine*) dominant in
pre–World War II America.[82] Second, the growing federal health

bureaucracy was increasingly preoccupied with the promises of laboratory and radiological research into the microbiological and anatomopathological aspects of infectious diseases, as opposed to the environmental or social behavioral factors that environmentalists assumed were dominant causes for the spread of these diseases.[83]

Third, an applied or technical form of multifactorialism—seroepidemiology and narrow epidemiology—was taking shape. This new applied epidemiology was exemplified best by Thomas Parran's policies and his so-called "Wassermann [test] dragnets." By employing mass seroepidemiology, the infectious disease research and control personnel of federal health agencies believed they now had the capacity to investigate the microbiological and "racial" determinants of epidemic disease, using large, presumably pure black and white populations. But, as we shall observe in a later section, black medical activists believed that seroepidemiology too frequently was viewed by federal health authorities (like Parran) as an end in itself. This led federal health authorities to bypass the task of trying to eliminate known environmental and social determinants for the disease's spread. Also ignored was the need to address racial segregation, which was widespread throughout the local- and state-run health bodies and public accommodations such as hospitals and sanitoriums.

By the mid-1930s, in order to move its anti-VD work and other field programs into black populations, the new federal health leadership followed the pattern set by local TB authorities in the preceding two decades. The heads of federal health agencies looked to the black physician, public health nurse, and community worker. Shortly after the 1930 White House Conference on Child Health, the Public Health Service assumed principal responsibility for providing facilities and operational resources to the National Negro Health movement. Prior to this incorporation, the tie between the Public Health Service and the Tuskegee-based Negro Health organization had been thin. In 1921 the Public Health Service began publishing the annual *Health Week Bulletin* for this organization; later, starting in 1927, it prepared annual posters. Before the early 1930s, the Negro Health organization's patchwork resources were donated primarily by black community-based organizations. Primary funders were the Annual Tuskegee Negro Conference sponsors, the National Negro Business League, the NMA, the National Negro Insurance Association, Tuskegee Institute, Howard University, and the Julius Rosenwald Fund (during the Negro Health organization's initial phase). Some support also came from state, county, and local departments of health, and a number of civic and voluntary health groups.[84]

During the Depression years, however, the Health Week organization came under great pressure to expand from growing numbers of state, county, and city constituencies interested in becoming participants. When the Public Health Service began administrating the organization from 1932 to 1934, a permanent director, offices and operating facilities were added. This enabled the Health Week organization to step up radically its local health awareness promotions. It began a new publication, the quarterly *National Negro Health News*, which became part of the nearly 200,000 pieces of health-awareness literature the organization circulated annually throughout black Americans communities[85] (see Table 4.1).

The Public Health Service's merger with the Negro Health movement was significant to New Deal health care policy specifically, and the modern history of national efforts to control epidemics in the urban black community generally for several reasons. First, it provided a communication bridge for the federal public health movement into the black lay community at the local, personal, household level. Nation-building and modernization, according to the classic communication theory of K. W. Deutsch, occurs among a population having "a community of shared meanings, or more broadly still, a group of people who have interlocking habits of communication."[86] Such communication entails not merely groups of people aggregating in the same space (for example, a town or city) at the same time, but also transaction flows, interaction patterns, that meld and integrate these people into a community.

During the Depression years, the transactional distance between federal health agencies and the nation's black community was substantial. If the emerging New Deal medical personnel, under the rousing leadership of Surgeon General Thomas Parran, was to have a national health movement, one that paid dividends to the nation-state in the form of a healthy, clear-minded, well-muscled workforce, the health predicament of blacks in the rural South and increasingly in the heart of the cities had to be addressed. As Parran remarked in his 1937 overview of black health problems, echoing Hoover's earlier health nationalism, "tax-payers [had] to prevent the spread of disease if only to avoid such economic losses as payments to men and women made unemployable by disease and maintenance of expensive institutions for the care of the sick and incapacitated."[87] Thus, this bridge enabled the anti–VD and TB campaigns, as well as other Public Health Service programs such as mass health surveys, and widening of maternal and infant care to proceed more effectively.

Besides closing the communication gap between the national

TABLE 4.1

Summary of the 1936 National Health Week Data

Number of States Participating	30
Number of Communities Participating	2,800

Clean-up:

Number of places (homes and lots)	65,100
Number of insect/rodent-control activities	35,015
Number of outhouses improved or constructed	8,100
Number of paint-up projects	3,750
Number of plant-and-flower projects	20,100
Number of clean-up activities not under other headings	18,250

Educational:

Number of lectures	3,832
Attendance	418,000
Number of radio talks	264
Number of pieces of literature distributed	160,310
Number of newspaper articles	1,017
Number of motion pictures	378
Attendance	82,500
Number of health exhibits	801
Attendance	33,500

Practical:

Number of clinics	750
Attendance	68,700
Number of plays, pageants, games, etc.	2,005
Attendance	121,250

Number of Local Prizes Awarded	191

Field Services (including preliminary and follow-up visits)

Number of states	6
Number of localities	13
Number of days	62
Number of organizations served	90
Number of lectures and conferences	221
Attendance	24,500
Number of motion pictures and exhibits	25
Attendance	10,315

Copies of literature distributed	9,250

Source: R. C. Brown, "The National Negro Health Week Movement," *JNE*, 6, no. 2 (July 1937): 561.

public health establishment and the black community, the Negro Health organization was a convenient instrument for the federal public health establishment to use to attempt transforming the inner health values of common black folk. Only when blacks had accepted the cultural authority of the physician and modern medical treatment could they be expected to attend clinical programs.[88] During the 1920s great numbers of Americans had been impressed by the physician and hospital care that they were receiving with increasing regularity. Moreover, the middle class was bombarded with popular health literature published by medical and public health professions. Magazines such as *Hygeia* (published by the American Medical Association) and *The Nation's Health* (American Public Health Association) "disseminate[d] the gospel of personal hygiene and scientific medicine," according to medical historian Victoria Harden. The result of these public relations efforts "was a growth of positive feeling for public health measures, scientific medicine, and scientific research [which] quickly permeated the fabric of American life."[89]

But the movement to popularize the medical profession and the medical scientific approach to personal health had had little attractiveness to the masses of African-Americans during the 1920s and Depression years. A folk health system interlacing Afro-Christian religious world-views, an abundance of dynamic faith and women healers, the omnipresent black spiritual church, and magical belief, were still powerful forces in urban black working-class communities, North and South.[90] Further, as late as 1937 over one-half of the more than 250,000 black infants born yearly were still delivered by midwives, including one-forth of those born in southern cities and one-third in northern cities.[91] Even the most dedicated physicians serving black community clientele felt at times overwhelmed with despair by lay blacks' energetic devotion to their folk healers, spiritualists, and the like. In an address in 1934 Dr. Peyton F. Anderson, president of the Central Harlem Medical Society, called for a "war against these parasites":

> Among the medical problems which impose a curse upon our group in this section [of the city] is the charlatan or quack or medical trickster. Why should some 150 physicians stand by and see our people swindled of their money and debased mentally and injured physically by fakirs, be they of the religious-mystic type or of any other type? When we have sufficiently protested the criminal activities of the prescribing barber, the counter prescribing druggist, the voodooist, the Indian herb root quacks,

the snake charming medicine crook, the evil spiritualists who
attempt healing, the hypnotists, the mental healers—all of
which infest our community to an extent that is far beyond our
individual appreciation.[92]

Thus, immersed in a fluctuating cultural and folk-healing world that
blended agrarian, African, and spiritualist ingredients; trapped at the
nation's socioeconomic bottom; and segregated from most of the
nation's mainstream public health and physician resources, the cultural movement to exalt scientific medicine was initially of little
importance to typical urban black communities.

By 1937 Thomas Parran believed that health consciousness
among blacks in recent years had been rising, but not high enough.
In his anti-VD programs, Parran maintained that in the paternal
South, the black masses trusted whites—"except where he [the
black] has suffered from sharp dealing and has good reason to be
suspicious"—and also government doctors. But he stressed that
black people's cultural bond was impenetrable without black health
workers or civic leaders laying the groundwork.

The Negro trusts the elders of his own race. Their older generation has an influence with the young that is far greater than
among us [whites]. He trusts the educated man and woman of
his race; except, again, when he has suffered from some
attempt of theirs to take advantage of his lack of education. The
negro preacher, the school-teacher, the occasional doctor are
the acknowledged leaders of their race. Arrangements were
made through them for talks in the schools and churches.[93]

Parran was buoyed by the involvement of the black community in the
new, federalized National Health Week movement: "The Negro has
shared in this dissemination of health information through agencies
of both white and colored origin and direction." But, to his thinking,
blacks were taking just the first steps toward recognizing the supremacy of modern medical science. "In the light of truth, as opposed
to superstition, dogma, and exploitation," Parran stated, the black
American "is becoming more intelligent concerning health matters in
general and his own status in particular. He is more alert to and active
in the requirements for control of his health problems, protection of
his home and community in which he lives, and prolongation of a life
of service and security for himself and his people."[94]

The Negro Health Week program also amplified the broader

political arguments that Parran and other New Deal public health strategists used to rationalize the higher death and illness rates of blacks. Public health planners would rely on these ideas in later decades when addressing health crises of black American communities. Meliorism was one such idea; that is, the notion that black America's health, like that of the nation's general citizenry, was mainly improving, no matter how bad local black medical professionals or community workers perceived their specific community's health problems to be.

The Parran strategists also emphasized nation-state authority as the chief instrument for promoting public health. This approach stressed that the state governmental units, coordinated by a centralized, federal regulatory body, was the most effective instrument to plan and implement health movements throughout black communities. It ruled out health care policy derived from civilian voluntary movements nurtured within black communities and lay institutions (and, conceivably, aligned with other medical care sectors). Parran made this clear in an 1937 overview of the Public Health Service and blacks: "The Negro has both opportunities and responsibilites inherent in the complex problem of his health status and the challenging need of its effective solution. However, the immediate responsibility for the future development of programs for the conservation of Negro health undoubtedly *rests with the states* and the communities within the states."[95]

With lines into the black community opened via the black public health sector and the lay Negro Health movement, Thomas Parran moved to nationalize the anti-VD drive. He viewed syphilis as "an epidemic disease [which] is kept alive, and spreads in the population by a series of small epidemics."[96] Thus, the programmatic approach by Public Health Service under Parran, and passed down to state and local health officials, centered on seroepidemiological sweeps to unearth serial or "localized" outbreaks. Mass serological testing was encouraged of populations considered at high risk for infections, such as persons arrested for sex offenses and vagrancy. The follow-up tasks, so-called contact tracing, had been modeled after the case-finding method long used in earlier anti-TB campaigns. Contact tracing involved identification of individuals suspected of having had contacts with a clinically infected carrier. Ultimately, this form of "sole-leather epidemiology" would yield the source of the case's infection and also that of individuals who may have been infected by the case brought to treatment. Finally, Parran employed the power of mass publicity and the authoritative rings of government pronoucements to try to deter social conduct influential in spreading this communicable disease.[97]

5

The actual results of the anti-VD operations by the Public Health Service throughout the nation's urban black communities were, by the close of the 1930s, viewed appreciatively by most black health leaders and white physician-researchers with close ties to the black medical profession. But this group also cautioned against overestimating both the scientific results and public health benefits to black Americans as a whole. First, the diagnostic findings of the mass serologic surveys conducted by the Public Health Service were of insignificant interpretive value for urban black (or, for that matter white) populations. The first round, in 1929–31, of the service's mass surveys (in cooperation with the Rosenwald Fund) involved Wassermann tests of some 35,000 people, but took in place in rural areas of six southern states.[98] In 1932 the infamous Tuskegee Syphilis Study (TSS) was commenced in Macon County, Alabama, involving 400 infected and 200 uninfected black men as controls. It is well documented that TSS became one of the worst breaches of medical ethics of contemporary times. A recent panel of medical and federal government experts on regulation of human experimentation reviewed TSS. It held that "the Public Health Service Study of Untreated Syphilis in the Male Negro in Macon County, Alabama, was ethically unjustified [even] in 1932."[99]

As late as 1937 H. H. Hazen, the prominent Howard University medical professor, still questioned the use of patchy epidemiological data from, for example, specific hospitals, obstetrical services, and 1920 army medical records, to infer the syphilis incidence of larger black populations, much less the entire black American "race." Almost all of this incidence data had been collected on small sets of what he termed a "hospital class" of blacks: general hospital patients with a variety of illnesses, or patients of obstetrical and pediatric clinics. Moreover, the sensitivity and specificity of the serologic tests could be substantially inaccurate, depending on the quality of the laboratory and serologic test. Even the Wassermann tests gave a significant proportion of false positive results and was eventually discontinued. Thus, Hazen believed these earlier data on the prevalence of syphilis among blacks (and whites) could be serious overestimates; and certainly they offered very little comparative statistics on prevalence of syphilis *within* various black occupational groups.[100]

Also around this time Julian H. Lewis, of the University of Chicago and Provident Hospital, described the effort in the medical scientific community to "fix at some numerical level the amount of syphilis among colored people" as an exercise in futility. The methods used spanned "from pure guesses to the Wassermann testing of whole communities," he observed, and "estimates of the prevalence of syphilis in Negroes have ranged from 12 to 74.1 percent." He and other critics of the research data on black syphilis rates attributed this biostatistical chaos to "imperfections in serological tests, lack of uniformity in technics used, the number of tests made on each individual, variations in the age, sex, marital status, number, geographical distribution, and, most of all, the socio-economic level of the different groups [that] profoundly affect the results."[101]

As for the Rosenwald Fund–Public Health Service's surveys in the black South, these too could generate gross fallacies when extrapolated to determine syphilis incidence onto the general black population. Lewis found the Public Health Service studies:

> represent no more than what they are: namely surveys of a particular class of Negroes in communities which, unfortunately, are characteristic of many parts of the deep South and which for the most part are made up of ignorant, oppressed, uninhibited sharecroppers on cotton plantations among whom syphilis varies with the degree of physicial and financial victimization by plantation owners and the availability of treatment facilities.[102]

The most accurate data on the black urban–rural syphilis incidence did not appear until 1942 when studies were done on nearly 1.9 million inductees and volunteers for World War II.[103]

In the area of resources for VD treatment and testing, no uniform national program emerged to provide resources for the urban black poor presumably heavily hit by the disease. Before 1936 only a jumble of resources packaged individually by medical institutions and local public health programs had developed. Municipal and black hospitals in large cities had to develop their own syphilis testing and treatment facilities throughout the early and mid-1930s. Each institution used various combinations of public funds (local, state, or federal) to start or enlarge their own syphilis services or clinics. But these services were frequently too limited or the patients had insurmountable personal circumstances that interrupted their treatment.

In New York City, for instance, Harlem Hospital did not have the resources to treat all of the syphilis cases that applied for treatment. When Shirley W. Wynne, the commissioner of health, investigated the matter (in the winter of 1933–34) she also found "a large proportion of [the hospital's] patients have become delinquent because the majority are almost penniless and lack the necessary carfare."[104] Other examples of municipal or black hospitals that handled with some effectiveness poor blacks in need of VD testing or treatment included Hubbard Hospital in Nashville, and Flint-Goodridge Hospital in New Orleans (funded by the Public Health Service or state board of health). Each screened patients for syphilis free of charge. When funds were available, Flint-Goodridge supplied the necessary pharmaceuticals also without charge.[105]

As soon as Parran became surgeon general and managed to get wide publicity for his nationwide anti-VD program, black physicians sought to support the drive. "[A]fter we heard that the Surgeon General had taken such a manly stand in this [VD] program," Dr. G. W. Bowles, an NMA official from Pennsylvania recounted, "[w]e started to communicate with the Public Health Service. I personally wrote several letters to the Public Health Service offering the services of the organized Negro [physician] group of this country toward a solution of this problem."[106] The NMA became the first national organization to vote to cooperate officially with the syphilis control campaign of the Public Health Service.[107] During the summer of 1936 it established its Commission on the Eradication of Syphilis composed of twelve physicians. Using the anti-VD programs of the black public health center in Norfolk as its model, throughout the late 1930s and early 1940s, the Commission reported, "Colored physicians in urban and rural districts of the South are organizing small laboratories and clinics [but] [u]nfortunately, while the number of Negro clinics is increasing, they as yet represent but a fraction of the number needed, particularly in the deep South."[108]

Following the growth in federal funds for VD control programs triggered by the Social Security (1935) and Lafollette–Bulwinkle (1938) Acts, urban black communities did gain concretely. From 1938 to 1940 clinical facilities for VD treatment increased nationwide from 1,750 to nearly 3,000. Expansion of testing and treatment in the southeastern states over roughly this same timespan also led to substantial increases in the number of VD cases identified and blacks entering treatment, as well as an overall decline in syphilis rates.[109] But despite the black medical community's eagerness to participate in the government's anti-VD movement, this growth did not reach the level expected either by them or their white medical-specialist allies like Ornstein and Hazen.

Other federal agencies less immersed in medical scientific issues carried out quite effective public health programs for the nation's poor blacks. Equally, if not more effective than the United States Public Health Service, but not given much attention in the history of American public health during the New Deal, were the black community health projects of the Works Progress Administration (WPA). This agency served as an important wing and funder of the federal government's work to survey illness and infectious disease throughout black American communities and to expand public health programs for this population. Usually coordinated with the Public Health Service, WPA projects focused on promoting health services and publicity campaigns at the local level. It provided personnel and organization in programs for venereal disease and TB control, as well as other diseases such as typhus fever, trachoma, and malaria, and community health problems including infant and maternity care, and sanitation.[110]

The WPA also coimplemented mass studies of American health that included health conditions of black populations, serving as a primary funder for the 1935–36 National Health Survey. A project of the Public Health Service, the National Health Survey became one of the largest national morbidity studies of the twentieth century.[111] Unlike the Public Health Service, however, whose policies for blacks during and immediately after the survey became centered mostly on anti-VD campaigns and demonstration projects throughout the black South, the WPA was more diversified and encouraged flexible roles for lay blacks.

The WPA's anti-TB work, for instance, involved largely data collection throughout black communities where the disease was suspected of having great impact. The data were then used by local and state authorities to campaign for more medical care facilities for black TB victims. By 1937 WPA workers had conducted TB surveys in more than ten states. When the WPA's surveys uncovered one of the highest concentrations of TB in the black community of Washington, D.C., the agency followed up by assisting in expansion or reconstruction of treatment facilities in local hospitals as well as the erection of a new sanitorium for children with TB located in Glenn Dale, Maryland. In Jacksonville, Florida, the WPA worked jointly with the local county Tuberculosis Association and city authorities and built a fifty-bed rest home for black patients. The WPA also built a brick building for a TB clinic in Macon, Georgia that served both blacks and whites.[112]

As for VD control, the WPA served as an extension of the Public Health Service's efforts to expand the use of health personnel and clinics in black and white neighborhoods. It trained workers to assist in making Wassermann tests, conducted surveys to establish the incidence of syphilis and gonorrhea, organized the referral of VD patients to local hospitals for treatment, and staffed clinics operated in evenings for those unable to attend regular facilities during day hours. A WPA assessment of its own work in 1937, in fact, illustrates that the racial focus had been established by the Public Health Service while the WPA put concrete programs in motion:

> Some of these [WPA-assisted VD] clinics were established especially for colored patients, and staffed in part by colored workers, in recognition of the discovery of the Public Health Service that the prevalence of venereal disease is higher among colored patients than among white. Many factors responsible for this condition—such as the social and economic status of the patients, their access to treatment facilties, and their failure to realize the seriousness of the disease and the necessity for early and adequate treatment—have been changed by the establishment of active clinics in Negro districts and by the increased effort to locate—and to bring in for examination and treatment if necessary—all infected persons.[113]

That clinical-service projects for the few could substantially change the socioeconomic situation and public awareness of these diseases among the many, was, of course, an overstatement. Nonetheless, this remark is evidence of the power that federal officials and public health workers now attributed to the environmental medical paradigm; and of the WPA's integral role in implementing specific, community-based health services for needy black areas.

Between 1935 and 1937 WPA projects throughout the South had certainly enhanced Public Health Service and local public agency campaigns against malaria, typhoid fever, dysentery, hookworm, and other diseases associated with poor sanitation and rural poverty. Throughout the century malaria had been a leading cause of morbidity and death worldwide. Endemic to regions of Asia, Africa, and Central and South America, malaria is a parasitic disease spread primarily where the mosquito vectors are persistent. It was learned in the early 1900s, largely through systematic mosquito control measures initiated by Col. William Gorgas in the Canal Zone, that the prevalence of malaria could be substantially reduced.[114] During the mid-1930s, WPA workers constructed drainage ditches, and filled in swampy areas and sluggish streams, gradually reducing mosquito concentrations responsible for spreading the disease. In 1937 the Surgeon General credited such WPA projects as having done more in three years to reduce malaria risks facing millions of Americans than had been accomplished during the four prior decades.[115]

Another aspect of WPA's health work within black communities involved urban areas. One WPA project that directly lowered disease prevalence was its campaign against typhus fever throughout Chicago's South Side, one of the nation's largest black communities. WPA staff worked jointly with the United States Department of Agriculture and the Public Health Service in projects to exterminate rodents and control this disease. Especially deadly, typhus fever can kill more than half its victims depending on such cofactors as age, nutritional conditions, concurrent diseases, and probably prior exposure. Vital to epidemic typhus is infected lice and louse feces spread by rats. The WPA workers helped expand the use of simple hygienic procedures such as rat control, bathing, and laundering of clothes and bedding.[116]

Other agencies that played a significant role in broadening visibility of black American health problems was the Children's Bureau (of the United States Labor Department) and the Public Works Administration (PWA). After the passage of the Social Security Act, the Children's Bureau stepped up its surveys and research on maternal and infant health. It also provided support through state health departments to expand child health and welfare services. The Bureau's surveys on infant and maternal mortality sought to raise awareness among public health and political officials of the serious problems blacks faced in these areas. Especially hard-hitting were the surveys of one of its senior statisticians, Elizabeth C. Tandy. In 1937 she estimated that about 22,000 or 8.8 percent of the roughly 250,000 black babies born each year died before age one. Moreover, 2,400 black women had died annually during 1933–35, proving that "[d]iseases of pregacy and childbirth were responsible for the deaths of more Negro women [aged 15–44 years] than any other disease except tuberculosis." Her studies indicated time and time again that a substantial proportion of these deaths of black mothers and infants could be prevented with proper prenatal and natal care.[117]

The Children's Bureau also assisted a number of states in developing maternal and infant care services as well as a few demonstration prenatal clinics for their cities and counties heavily populated by needy blacks. Adhering to the policy that black medical personnel could best serve the nation's needy black communities, given the social and cultural race segregation, the Bureau helped states furnish postgraduate education or courses for a few black physicians to improve their pediatric, obstetrical, and public health skills, as well as teach new skills to their local colleagues. Also, groups of black midwives received training in states where they were in large numbers by trained nurse-midwives. Finally, the Bureau employed a black social worker with whom state agencies could consult on matters pertaining to homeless or dependent black children.[118] In the meanwhile, the PWA, either through direct assistance or loans, provided more than 8,000 hospital beds in 17 southern states for blacks.[119]

6

Throughout the New Deal era, the social and professional activism of black doctors, nurses, and allied professionals intensified markedly. Generally, their dissatisfaction was part of the rise in militant consciousness throughout the rank-and-file urban black community. As the international crisis of Euronationalism and race sharpened, so did the racial caste at home. Declassed northern and southern whites, suffering the pain and frustration of the economic collapse, intensified social segregation as they fought to retain their share of local power and social authority. "The New Deal has actually changed the whole configuation of the Negro problem," Gunnar Myrdal observed. "Until then the practical Negro problem involved civil rights, education, charity, and little more. Now it has widened, in pace with public policy in the new 'welfare state,' and involves housing, nutrition, medicine, education, relief and social security, wages and hours, working conditions, [and] child and woman labor."[120]

With the political and social agitation among blacks elevating nationwide, black medical professionals became especially active in the National Association of the Advancement of Colored People (NAACP), the nation's major civil rights organization, but also in the newer, more aggressive National Negro Congress (NNC). The latter organization tried to coordinate a national network of black community organizations and leaders. At its initial meeting in Chicago, representatives from more than 500 community-work agencies and civic groups attended. Under the leadership of A. Philip Randolph, its early president, the NNC organized local councils and mass meetings to further economic and political equality for blacks. In 1936 more black doctors (nine) than attorneys (five) were on the NNC's presiding committee. Two black physicians, Charles A. Lewis of Philadelphia and Robert A. Simmons of Massachusetts, were among the Congress's six vice-presidents in 1938. When the NNC issued its resolutions growing from its national conference of October 1937, one dealt specifically with health. The health resolution stressed that the NNC "is keenly conscious of the intimate relation between Health and the Economic and Social Welfare of the people." It called for the expansion of maternity and child health care, as well as hospital facilities generally for blacks. It further urged that unemployment relief include food, dental care, eyeglasses, and medicines, and that black representatives sit on the planning committees of all government and private health agencies.[121]

Black medical leadership criticized federal and local health and relief agencies for their failure to put a substantial dent in the TB and infant mortality rates among blacks. The New Deal–era federal health and relief machinery had made some progress, distributing or stimulating small increments of direct relief, health facilities, and public health services througout black communities. But the overall health picture for blacks improved little, as did the employment, specialty training, or participation of black doctors, nurses and social welfare workers within the technological, educational and hospital-clinical structures of the country. Black medical leaders had come to believe the federal government throughout the New Deal had only given a hodgepodge of medical resources to (a) lessen the more obvious emergency health conditions in black communities ravaged by the Depression; and (b) to mobilize blacks for mass examination and treatment projects of the Public Health Service with its fever-pitch anti-VD campaigns.

Black medical professional associations, most notably the National Association of Colored Graduate Nurses (NACGN) as well as members of its national Advisory Council, criticized New Deal medical policy towards blacks. The Advisory Council was established in 1938 to increase support for educational and employment opportunities of black nurses generally, and other medical goals of black Americans. The chair of the Council was Ruth L. Roberts, board director for such organizations as the New York Tuberculosis Association and the National YWCA. The vice chair was Dr. Midian Bousfield, the Rosenwald Fund representative. Membership of the interracial Advisory Council included nearly sixty prominent medical, welfare, educational, and civic leaders such as publicist Claude Barnett, Louis T. Wright, nursing leaders Ella Best and Alma Haupt, and the prominent sociologists George Edmund Haynes and Charles S.

Johnson. The Council also had some notable white members such as the medical planner Michael M. Davis and Mrs. Thomas H. Parran.[122]

In 1937 and again in 1939 the first and second National Conference on the Problems of the Negro and Negro Youth convened in Washington, D.C. Organized under the auspices of President Roosevelt and with Mary McLeod Bethune as general secretary, these meetings were for developing recommendations for the racial policies and programs of the federal executive and legislative branches.[123] The Committee on Health and Housing within the National Conference, chaired by Dr. Bousfield, worked closely with Advisory Council members and developed a broad agenda relating to medical care and public health it wanted the federal government to address. At the 1939 Negro Youth Conference, Advisory Council members expressed dismay about the lack of progress on their numerous recommendation for improving the pressing health and medical training problems of black Americans. The nine priorities the Advisory Council and the Conference's Committee on Health and Housing had stressed were:

1. Better medical care and preventive medicine for the colored masses, utilizing fully additional funds made available under the Social Security Act.
2. The training and use of competent Negro personnel in health programs.
3. Internships and residence in hospitals for special training.
4. Additional public health nurses.
5. Greater financial support for Freedmen's Hospital and the Medical School of Howard University.
6. The use of Federal funds for the establishment of health centers in Negro neighborhoods under competent Negro staffs.
7. Use of Federal funds in the construction of more hospitals for Negroes.
8. The opening up of Veteran's Hospitals to Negro veterans and the inclusion of Negro doctors and nurses on these hospital staffs.
9. Freer use of Negro personnel in the program for crippled children under the Children's Bureau.

But between 1937 when these Conference recommendations had been delivered to government officials and the second conference in 1939, the federal government made virtually no improvements. In 1939 the conferees reported that except for progress in the syphilis treatment program, "there has been no notable change in the approach to Negro health problems." Two black physicians had been added (as associate medical officers) to the Division of Venereal Diseases Units, and the employment of black public health nurses had increased slightly. New York City received sufficient federal funds to construct a health center in a black residential area. But other cities, like Washington, D.C., in dire need of such centers, went wanting, even though "[t]uberculosis and infant mortality rates among Negroes in the District of Columbia still rank among the highest in the United States." While some federal money had come for hospital construction, it was only for shoring up segregated white-controlled hospitals or the usually substandard black hospitals. During 1938 about seven million dollars was expended "in the construction of Negro wings or Negro hospitals." North Carolina, Maryland, and Tennessee received $1.5 million to provide sanitoriums for blacks.[125]

Black Americans' sociomedical or health paradigm was not only a public, political stance for comprehensive medical care. It also encompassed an intellectual, scientific critique leveled by black medical activists in academic and policy–expert circles, a critique that grew throughout the post–World War II decades. According to the black health paradigm, equally threatening to the efforts for adequate medical care were the sociological and reputedly clinical theories and data (that is, racialist or multifactorial sociomedical constructions) postulating (or implying) genotypical race traits as an primary cause for higher black mortality from TB, syphilis and other diseases.

For example, in the winter of 1938–39 Abraham Stone, the editor of the *Journal of Contraception* asked Louis T. Wright to review Holmes's *The Negro's Struggle for Survival.* Shortly after, Wright sent Stone a blistering commentary on the book. According to Wright, Holmes misused isolated or erroneous medical facts to build an apparently medical-sociological verification of the black susceptibility argument. Holmes "stated that the skin of the Negro was thicker than the skin of white people." But according to Wright, "[a]s a surgeon who has operated on thousands of whites and Negroes, the fact is that all races vary in the degree of thickness of their skin, and even individuals *within* the same race do likewise." Wright excoriated Holmes' study, because Holmes "steps out of his field, as a biologist, to contradict authorities in [modern surgery and] other fields." Wright declared that "Professor Holmes' misstatements of fact . . . remove this book from the realm of scientific investigation. Pseudoscientific books and papers have long been used for propaganda purposes."[126]

In the upcoming chapters, we follow the interplay of the black relationist paradigm with the black community's changing structure and social movements for health improvement, and the nation's dominant medical establishment. It is the relationship between these three domains—the black health care sector, larger social change impulses emanating from the black community, and the institutional and intellectual character of American medicine—that will determine the efficacy of the various sociomedical responses to the current AIDS epidemic in black America.

Chapter 5

The Black Health Paradigm Solidifies:
From World War II to Pharmacological Revolution

As America mobilized industrially and militarily during World War II, a frenzy to guard what government leaders called the "health defense of the Nation" also erupted. Politicians, public health authorities, and business and philanthropic leaders all stressed that higher health and nutrition standards must be national priorities if the United States was to triumph over Hitlerism. This new health patriotism intensified government and voluntary efforts to control major diseases, especially venereal disease and TB. Recruitment required physical exams of millions of white and black Americans. As this screening reaffirmed that blacks suffered disproportionately from these diseases, national voluntary health organizations sought to rekindle the black public health superstructure and community activism to assist their efforts.

When the war years receded, however, so did the infatuation with the idea that the broad health status of blacks could be improved to equal that of whites. The continued overconcentration of TB, venereal disease, and infant and maternal mortality in black populations, coupled with ongoing shortages and segregation in medical facilities, professions and educational institutions, compelled black health activists to focus increasingly on advocating health care policies based on their own relationist epidemic paradigm. This health policy view gained even greater momentum among black medical leadership as American health care adjusted to the nation's growing central-city black populations.

Following World World War II, black medical and social welfare leaders joined the resurgent movement for national health insurance, which they believed was the only effective long-term solution to excess black mortality. But during the Cold War and Civil Rights eras, hopes for national health insurance faded from the domestic agenda. Black medical and social welfare leaders abandoned the

goal of universal access to medical care. In keeping with their relationist epidemic paradigm, they initially stressed more medical services for fighting the traditional communicable diseases. But during
the civil rights years, black health leadership focused more on
obtaining hospital services suitable for the broad range of health
problems concentrating in central-city black neighborhoods, and on
expanding the supply of black medical professionals to serve this
population.

Paralleling the black health community's heightened group
identity and broad view of disease was the rise of mainstream
medicine's effective pharmaceuticals for treating TB and venereal
diseases. These new medical weapons profoundly reversed the
destruction that major communicable disease had on the American
population. But these new treatments did not address directly other
disease crises black health leaders perceived to be raging in the
black communities. The historic and continuing division between
these two sociomedical currents—one, embracing multifactorial specialism (so-called scientific medicine); the other, interrelating clinical
and socioeconomic factors to explain and remedy sickness in the
individual black as well as the black community generally—largely
shaped the dominant issues regarding the control and elimination of
AIDS in the black American community.

1

Through the Second World War mortality of blacks, particularly
associated with infectious diseases as well as infant and maternal
mortality, continued to outdistance those of whites. While TB and
other major infectious diseases were declining throughout the general American population, black mortality from these ailments
remained relatively high, especially within black urban and youth
populations. Nationally, the death rate from TB dropped from nearly
150 per 100,000 in 1918 to 40 per 100,000 in 1945. From 1938 to
1939 black TB mortality rose in New York City from 949 deaths to
1,036. In numerous other major cities, blacks were more than one-
half of those dead from TB in 1939. That year blacks suffered 50
percent of the TB deaths in Baltimore; 58 in New Orleans; 72 in
Washington, D.C.; 78 in Birmingham; 78 in Atlanta; and 79 in Memphis. Nationally, blacks suffered 5,925 deaths or 32 percent of the
TB deaths reported in the nation's 46 largest cities.[1]

TB was an especially frequent killer of younger blacks. From
1940 to 1942 it was the leading cause of mortality for blacks aged 15

to 34, killing an average 3,700 of these young people yearly. From 1939 to 1940 the percentage of deaths among blacks due to TB aged 15 to 29 was extraordinarily high and reversed the trends toward decline of prior decades. In 1940 nearly one-third (29.2 percent) of the deaths of black male youths aged 15 to 19, and one-half (49.2) of the deaths of black females of that age group were caused by TB.[2]

Because TB was a declining national menace for white Americans, national health authorities now conceptualized TB as in a "residual stage," declining and pooling into "reservoirs" among racial minorities. One of the earliest, most influential health authorities enunciating this idea was Louis Dublin. In his address "The Mortality from Tuberculosis Among the Race Stocks in the Southwest," delivered before the 1941 annual meeting of the National Tuberculosis Association (NTA) held in San Antonio, Texas, Dublin stressed that the hidden frontier facing the NTA was "in various parts of the country [where] there are areas and groups, both large and small, among whom the control of tuberculosis is still in a very rudimentary state." He gave a general ethnic geography of TB in the Southwest. In Louisiana the high TB rate was caused by the disproportionately high population of black tuberculars there; in Texas, it was the Mexican and the black. For New Mexico and Arizona, the highest TB rates were among the Mexicans but also the mixed-Indian and "full-blooded" Indians. In California, "the resident tuberculosis problem is concentrated chiefly among the Mexicans, but there are sizable numbers of Chinese, Japanese and Filipinos, among whom the disease is widespread and fatal."[3]

But Dublin underscored that throughout the Southwest and the nation overall, blacks composed the largest concentration of tuberculars. "In the large, Negroes constitute the last great reservoir of tuberculosis in our country. They are responsible for over one quarter of all [TB] deaths." In Houston and San Antonio, the black TB mortality rate (about 138 per 100,000) was nearly three and one-half times greater than that of whites in these cities (about 40 per 100,000). Moreover, because the Southwest contained about 15 percent of the United States's black population, NTA officials and programs in this region must expect to "bear its share of the work and responsibility of solving this part of the tuberculosis problem."[4]

Alongside the TB crisis in black America stood the continuing venereal disease threat. The great shifts in the domestic population, loosening in social relations, and build-up in military personnel and installations conducive to promiscuity created the context for a rise in venereal disease during the early years of World War II. Nationally, syphilis rates for blacks in 1940 were estimated to be five times greater than those of whites.[5] But Thomas Parran and the Public Health Service, using Selective Service serologic reports for the first 2,000,000 selectees through 1943, estimated that syphilis among black men examined by Selective Service was actually ten times the rate of white men.[6]

Venereal disease prevalence in the black residential districts of major cities was also among the nation's highest. In New York City officials and medical experts began tabulating the health defects among those black and white recruits rejected for military service. Medical posts for the Selective Service had been set up throughout dozens of hospitals and health centers in New York City, staffed by some 1,100 doctors. The medical defects for New York's rejected recruits as a whole were compared with those of Selective Service posts in city sections that examined 60 to 99.8 percent blacks. This 1941 survey disclosed that rejections for blacks were substantially higher for disorders related to venereal disease, respiratory ailments, and heart diseases.[7] In Atlanta, where blacks made up nearly one-third of the city's roughly 500,000 total population, from 1942 to 1946 about 28,900 black residents, compared to only 8,000 whites, were reported by health officials to have syphilis or gonorrhea.[8]

Some medical investigators of venereal disease control tried to inform as well as shock when they described the crisis level these diseases had reached among city blacks. In 1946 two medical researchers studying venereal disease in Harlem throughout the war years cautioned that "colorful Harlem [social life] has been more vividly described and more widely read of than the Harlem of economic hardships and dreaded diseases." The researchers called this stretch of neighborhoods New York City's "largest venereal-disease–infested area." They pointed out that although it contained only 11 percent of Manhattan's population, "Harlem has: by disease, 33 percent of all cases of syphilis, and 44 percent of all cases of gonorrhea; by age groups, 57.6 percent of all infection in teen-age girls, and 45.4 percent of all infection in teen-age boys."[9]

Within each black community, the frequent infectious disease–related deaths and illness were witnessed painfully by the families of the stricken, neighbors, churches, and local family physicians. In turn, black medical leaders were angered that the nation's larger medical and political community seemed unconcerned. For example, in 1942 Dr. William A. Beck, a professor at Meharry Medical College, spoke about the black TB crisis on a radio show in Charleston, West Virginia. He pointed out that TB was still the second leading cause of deaths for blacks, and that there were about 250,000 active cases among blacks as well as an equal number of "silent cases." Dr. Beck asserted that programs throughout the nation to control TB in the black population would be doomed unless treatment and hospital facilities were made equally available to blacks and whites. He stressed that the "Negro physicians are pleading to hospital boards, hospital administrators, health officers, public spirited citizens, and to the great medical profession of these United States of America, for permission—in a larger measure—to acquire adequate knowledge and training, so that we may help to stop tuberculosis which is the axis enemy here in America."[10]

Dr. George D. Cannon, a prominent New York–area black physician and health coordinator for a Harlem grass-roots group on neighborhood problems, also condemned the TB epidemic in this community. Speaking on a popular black community radio program one day in 1946, Cannon called TB a plague among blacks. In New York City, he pointed out, the black TB mortality rate exceeded that of whites almost four and one-half times. Cannon emphasized that since 1942 about 1,000 blacks had died yearly from TB, to which the mayor, city health authorities, and national medical leaders were all but oblivious. In addition, private hospitals in the area were closing down:

> Here is a contagious disease [TB] killing people in the low income brackets at an outrageous rate yet health authorities don't get excited. Several days ago, a plane flew experts from Boston to Texas because of 5 children becoming ill with infantile paralysis—not a death but just becoming ill. They wanted to protect the other children. We in Harlem want protection too, not from just a paralyzed limb but from death itself. Should one serious contagious disease be treated different from another, from diphtheria, from typhoid, or smallpox?[11]

While Cannon commended the local public health clinic for having conducted some of the largest detection surveys for TB of any city health district, there remained a dire need for more hospital beds to isolate highly infectious TB cases. Cannon believed that cutting down the number of ambulatory infectious TB cases in neighborhood streets, boarding houses, etc., could help reduce mortality rates. He also urged that black physicians be brought into hospital TB services. "As its stands now," Cannon remarked, "there is not one practicing Negro physician on the visiting staff of a tuberculosis hospital in the city today or in the State of New York for that matter. And this despite the fact that this disease is the number one menace to their communities."[12]

In 1945–46 the General Education Board of the Rockefeller Foundation funded a major national survey to explore the health problems of urban blacks and ways to increase local preventive health programs in their communities. The National Urban League, in cooperation with the NTA, the National Organization of Public Health Nursing and the National Recreation Association investigated five major cities (three northern, two southern) with large black populations. The survey found that the most pressing medical problem was the shortage of VD clinics, hospital beds, and maternity, infant and child medical services for this population. After the survey by health and social welfare experts, the Urban League organized local councils composed of representatives from community social welfare agencies to provide health services most needed by these city's blacks.[13]

Prior to World War I municipal health authorities had been leery of involving black professionals in public health programs to control epidemics. While this policy was modified during the interwar decades, black health professionals were still usually limited to local projects or agencies. But during World War II and immediately after, national voluntary health agencies, especially the NTA and the American Social Hygiene Association (ASHA), quickly conferred with health and social welfare experts from black institutions to help plan and publicize these organizations' efforts to control disease in specific local black communities. The problem came when local health workers in black communities, despite their enthusiastic involvement as advisers and morale boosters, found public financial and medical resources wanting. Typical large medical institutions in the cities were geared toward applying the new powerful chemotherapies for treatment of TB and VD patients, than toward battling these ailments with preventive measures in the more complex social terrain of minority black communities.

As black and white venereal disease rates threatened to climb dramatically during the war years, the ASHA sought to expand the presence of black health professionals and community groups in the national anti–VD effort. The ASHA was a national health and welfare reform organization that focused on eliminating social ills such as venereal disease and prostitution. Both the ASHA and Public Health Service believed the black public health superstructure would be the most efficient means for bringing their public education campaign into black households, neighborhoods, schools, and military centers.[14]

The ASHA's national program targeted for black America was initiated in November 1943, by a conference held in cooperation with the Public Health Service and military medical units involved in venereal disease control.

The conference, titled "Negro Leaders On Wartime Problems in Venereal Disease Control," had been arranged discreetly by the ASHA and federal agencies specifically as a national "high-level" meeting to review the venereal disease problem of black Americans and to develop control programs. It was chaired by the dermatologist and Provident Hospital (Chicago) professor, Dr. T. K. Lawless, who had served on advisory committees to black affairs organized by the ASHA. Lawless was regarded highly throughout the black medical community as an academician, but also as a shrewd yet fair leader. Invitees to the meeting included other prominent black medical experts such as William A. Hinton and Paul B. Cornely, military officials and physician-officers, educational leaders like Mary McLeod Bethune, Jesse Jones, and Ambrose Caliver, and clerical heads of national black church organizations (see Appendix).

At the commencement of the ASHA's Negro Leaders conference, Lawless emphasized that "these diseases attack people without distinction as to race, creed, color or national origin, and must in turn be fought in the open by all people." But he also urged those in attendance to accept the reality that the nation's highest venereal disease rates rested in the "Negro population." Exploring the social and economic factors behind this pattern was one of the two central aims of the conference. The other conference theme was to look within the black community for solutions to this crisis. According to Lawless, "[t]he Negro should accept the opportunity and assume responsibility of contributing help and influence from within the race to the solution of the problem and the removal of whatever measure of stigma there is associated with it."[15]

The conference attendees separated their approach to the problem of venereal disease in the black community into three areas: (1) surveys of the medical prevalence of venereal diseases among blacks and sharing ideas on how best to publicize these facts throughout the black community; (2) ways to study more extensively the social conditions pervading black communities that lead to the spread of syphilis and the forms of social welfare resources needed to eliminate or minimize these conditions; and (3) studying the ways that official and voluntary agencies can assist "Negro voluntary organizations" on the local, state and federal levels.[16]

The ASHA conference resulted in a number of specific recommendations. A manual of facts about venereal disease was to be compiled and distributed to various organizations in the black community encountering venereal disease problems. It also recommended expanding the supply of black medical personnel in both the private practice and public health fields. Specific steps suggested included increasing enrollments at Howard and Meharry medical schools, expanding orientation courses on venereal disease problems for black community workers offered by the Public Health Service, and more postgraduate education on new technical aspects of recognizing and treating venereal disease for black medical personnel, particularly those located in the South. "The training of Negro personnel should not be limited to physicians only," the conference report stressed, "but should apply to all personnel that may be connected with this program, such as nurses, health educators, social workers and laboratory technicians."[17]

The social aspects behind the high venereal disease rates in black communities presented the most serious difficulties to prior and current anti-VD campaigns. The conference leaders pointed out that there were 3,800 centers for VD treatment throughout the country, but the centers were not arresting the spread of venereal disease throughout black populations because of various social factors. High venereal disease rates of blacks were largely the result of low wages and educational levels, as well as inadequate housing and lack of recreational facilities. Also, there was widespread social and legal disorder throughout black communities. Laws against commercialized prostitution went unenforced, and the practices and personnel of law agencies in black communities were generally deficient; all of which caused "a failure of law enforcement officials to practice a single standard of law enforcement . . . as related to Negro communities." Finally, the health care and social welfare leaders of white and black communities appeared genuinely unable to work together. Future anti-VD activities aimed at black communities, the conferees asserted, would have to overcome "[a]n attitude of defeatism toward the problems of venereal disease control on the part of many white community leaders and of frustration among leaders in the Negro community."[18]

From this conference and others organized shortly afterwards by the ASHA emerged practical ideas and programs for black community work. These programs attempted to tap the strong local lay and professional anti-VD interests growing throughout the nation's black communities, and weave them with state, federal, and philanthropic community-work resources. In 1945 the Association called upon government health agencies and the medical sector to provide wide roles for blacks in their anti-VD campaigns, setting forth these principles:

1. That Negro leadership and organization should be asked to assume the fullest responsibility for the promotion of such a program.
2. That the employment of Negro professional personnel in various phases of VD control programs should be expanded as rapidly as possible and that the opportunity for training Negroes for VD work sould be increased as rapidly as possible.
3. That the community at large, including public and private health agencies, should encourage, support, and cooperate with Negro efforts in every possible way.[19]

Anti-VD programs sponsored by ASHA for blacks took a variety of forms. Some were initiated by statewide associations of black welfare activists, as was the case in Houston. Others, such as those in St. Louis (Mo.), Nashville, Cincinnati, and Hartford (Conn.), were incorporated into existing municipal health agencies and citywide private charitable organizations. Finally, some ASHA programs for blacks were started from local organizations specifically planned to coordinate the anti-VD campaign. This was the approach followed in Battle Creek (Mich.) and Pensacola (Fla.).[20]

In the meantime, national voluntary health associations such as the NTA continued to build local community programs staffed by black personnel in cities throughout the country. These programs focused largely on public education activities such as radio programs and literature dissemination, clinics for preschool children, and student health institutes for high school and college youth. A few of the NTA projects in major cities were coordinated jointly with the Public Health Service, and focused on intensive diagnostic campaigns. In Harlem, for example, a TB case-finding survey by mass X-rays of 20,000 persons was conducted during 1945–46 under the auspices of the Harlem Committee.[21]

The overall approaches of major philanthropic health organizations and federal health agencies to eliminate venereal disease, TB, and other health problems in black communities, however, still had serious weaknesses. First, officials of the ASHA, NTA, and Public Health Service fully accepted state and local official agencies as the dominant authority for controlling and directing the financial and medical resources provided by the federal government.[22] But

innumerable black community populations in need of these disease-control resources faced Jim Crow political disfranchisement or
city machine politics. Such black populations were, in effect, alienated from the federal and state political apparatus upon which the
local public health care and hospital programs were engineered,
funded, distributed, and monitored. Further, the public health
infrastructure itself was not a well-endowed component of the
nation's medical establishment. In fact, during the 1950s and 1960s,
the number of public health professionals and local units changed
very little despite the explosion in the size and number of American
urban communities.[23]

The National Urban League's 1945–46 survey of black health
and medical resources in five large cities uncovered deeply rooted
problems in VD- and TB-control programs. Dr. Paul B. Cornely was
one of the study's black directors. Among the nation's most expert,
but at this time unsung, public health physicians, Cornely pinpointed
the survey's central observation: "Much has been said . . . about the
high prevalence of venereal diseases in the Negro, and yet in three of
these cities the venereal disease program was woefully inadequate,
the clinic facilities dilapidated and unattractive, one of these being in
an old city jail." In the largest city surveyed, which had a black population of 120,000, there was only one VD clinic for blacks.[24]

Thus, while national philanthropic and public health authorities
were able to cultivate a wide variety of advisory and field personnel
roles for black health and social work professionals and lay leaders—as Parran and the New Deal/Public Health Service programs
did during the 1930s—the official public health agencies at the state
level and below, as well as the mainstream medical institutions, usually segregated these black employees and consultants.[25] The traditional medical elite at the head of the nation's major medical
schools, hospitals, and federal health agencies retained sole authority to dictate to federal and state government the nature and scope
(or nonexistence) of epidemics in urban black America, as well as
the appropiate governmental response.

It was this medical infrastructure that decided for the larger
society what resources and funds should be available for prevention
and treatment, and the acceptibility of strategies to be used in campaigns to eliminate particular diseases or health problems in the
black community. Furthermore, this dominant medical research and
professional community determined, based on the epidemiological
paradigm they supported, perceptions of the direction of the epidemic threat, the populations most at risk and most amenable to

treatment; in short, the most worthwhile population and community that the body politic should assist.

Black advisers to the government and national charitable health agencies broadened lay America's view of the black community's health problems and capacity for group self-help. Nonetheless, the key officials and institutions in federal health agencies and national organized medicine were under no pressure to implement the medical and social welfare approaches suggested by this black health personnel. Writing in a 1943 issue of the Urban League's *Opportunity*, Pauline Coggs raised an early voice against the proliferation of race advisers in the Public Health Service and other federal agencies. These agencies "acknowledged the exclusion of the Negro from the normal stream of community and national life by employing Negro specialists to promote programs among Negroes to apprise the agency of the impact of social problems upon them." Furthermore, the Negro advisers "work within a specified field and are forced to rely on the inadequate machinery of state and local governments and [weak] Negro organizations for the prosecution of their objectives."[26]

During the 1950s and 1960s, black medical and welfare leadership deepened their unique health paradigm, merging their relational medical perception for the persistence of epidemic disease in black communities with their social and health policy activism. Meanwhile, the status quo leadership of the nation's medical care institutions were not compelled to bring the infectious disease crises facing black communities to center stage, especially since chemotherapeutic breakthroughs were reducing drastically the white American population's mortality from these diseases.

2

In the minds and activities of a growing number of post–World War II black medical leaders and white medical experts, the pattern of high disease rates found in black communities was determined neither primarily by biological-racial factors nor by unhealthy cultural attitudes presumed widespread in the black community. They stressed, instead, the heightened urbanization, political-racial discrimination, and material and medical deprivation blacks faced. During the 1940s and 1950s there was, indeed, an immense growth in the nation's central-city black population. The percentage of black Americans in the inner-city sections of metropolitan regions went from 14.5 in 1900, to 30.6 in 1930, to 51.5 in 1960.[27] Unlike prior periods, when intense episodes of mass migration from rural to urban, and North to South were largely responsible for the leap in urban black population, the surge in black city-dwellers during the 1940s through early 1960s was caused more by upward fertility and longer life-expectancy trends among urban black populations, as well as urbanization concentrated in the South that pulled in rural black residents of this region. Throughout both the northern and southern cities the proportion of the black population within the "dependent" age brackets (that is, below the age of 15 or over the age of 65), was significantly higher than that of whites; females, typically more needy of medical services due to their reproductive function, tended to outnumber males among the 1940s northern black migrant populations. Finally, a steady decline in black maternal and infant mortality occurred during 1945–65, due largely to the long-term effects of public health campaigns initiated in the New Deal and World War II periods.[28]

The increase in post–World War II America's black urban population, which tended to require more medical services because of age or gender, was coupled with rapid fragmentation of the traditional, spatially concentrated black residential/business communities of the cities. This fragmentation was a result of wide-ranging slum clearance and urban renewal programs initiated during the New Deal and World War II decades. The physical shattering of traditional inner-city black enclaves did not lead to assimilation of black residents into predominantly white sections, but merely reshaped or "verticalized" segregated housing patterns, as well as encouraged epidemiological denial in middle- and upper-class medical and residential sectors. Indeed, public housing projects in numerous ways actually reinforced a more insidious, economically based, racial discrimination in medical care. With the new public housing enclaves came a subtle "tilt" in broader metropolitan race relations that tended to lower the visibility or threat of epidemics affecting black project-dwelling populations.

First, "project" renewal concentrated low-income blacks together, while eliminating commercial buildings suitable for small shopkeepers, entrepreneurs and medical professionals. Through the 1940s family physicians had provided a flexible range of medical services in their homes or offices including "spot diagnosis," treatment for minor injuries, radiology for chest and small bones, minor surgery, advice on suspected psychiatric disturbances, and some obstetric and pediatric care.[29] But urban renewal not only destabilized poor blacks psychosocially by forcing their physical relocation, it also undermined the neighborly contact between these lower-income blacks and the traditional black family physician.[30]

Second, concentrating poorer blacks into project building complexes reduced substantially their contact with larger white populations of the metropolis. In prior decades blacks who may have had infectious diseases labored or lived in close proximity to urban whites. Thus, urban blacks were perceived by health authorites as capable of transmitting epidemics to a city's larger, white population as well. But with city housing patterns (and suburban white population growth) becoming more racially divided, there was no cause for general citywide alarm if an epidemic struck inside black city sections.

Third, when urban redevelopment accelerated the segregation of blacks by income and race, urban voluntary hospitals under predominantly white control simply relocated away from these high-rise, low-income black sections to avoid shouldering the extensive medical care required by this inner-city poor sector. They also denied privileges to black physicians in order to avoid serving the black patients of these black doctors. In New York City during 1948, for instance, the Hospital Council of Greater New York investigated affiliations of the city's 225 black physicians. Of 170 having some form of hospital staff appointment, just 49 were with voluntary hospitals; the rest were concentrated in municipal hospitals.[31] Moreover, most of the small number of black hospitals in large cities became increasingly isolated from black middle-class clientele, overburdened with treating the indigent, and destined to fail financially.[32]

Horace Cayton and St. Clair Drake described this process of urban black population growth and impoverishment in 1961 when they compared Chicago then, to the Chicago they had studied some sixteen years earlier in their famous *Black Metropolis*. Chicago's black population had almost doubled during the 1950–60 decade, going from 492,000 to 813,000, but only 60,000 had migrated from the South. Cayton and Drake emphasized that "[s]lum clearance and urban redevelopment programs have wiped out the concentrated cluster of [black] lower-class institutions and scattered the population. But as a sub-culture, the 'World of the Lower Class' still exists."[33]

The poverty and social isolation from adequate medical care experienced by the black inner-city, working-class populations were mirrored in their higher mortality rates from major diseases during the latter 1940s. While the national mortality rates for infant and maternal mortality, and communicable diseases declined precepitously both before and following World War II, such deaths still contributed substantially to the disproportionately higher black mortality through the 1940s. Health data compiled by Louis Dublin in 1949, still the nation's leading health statistician, revealed mortality from communicable diseases was substantially higher among the more than two million black policyholders of Metropolitan Life Insurance. He attributed this black–white mortality gap largely to traditional epidemic diseases that had declined in the nation's general population but still remained at menacing levels throughout black communities. Dublin found six causes of death most responsible for the black–white mortality gap: TB, pneumonia and influenza, nephritis, cerebral hemorrhage, syphilis, and homicide. "The principal item in this difference," he wrote, "is tuberculosis [which] was two and three-quarter times that for white males, while among females the ratio was almost four to one." Syphilis death rates were four and one-half times higher for black males than for white males, and six times higher for black females than for white females. Finally, maternal and infant death rates for blacks were double and triple those of whites, respectively.[34]

Given their higher fertility, mortality, and morbidity rates, as well as residential seclusion, the new urban black population of post–World War II America experienced critical shortages in medical services for maternity care, pediatrics, chronic illness, geriatric needs, and acute care. Dr. E. I. Robinson, the president of the National Medical Association (NMA), stated in 1946 that "[t]here is a lack of hospital facilities of all types for Negroes." He estimated that throughout the nation, the ratio of general-hospital beds available to blacks was only one-tenth to one-half the ratio of beds allocated to whites. In the South about 10,000 blacks died annually from TB but their were fewer than 6,000 hospital beds available for black Southern residents, some 25,000 beds short of the number recommended by the American Public Health Association.[35]

Black medical and social welfare strategists like Dr. Robinson in the years during and shortly following World War II tended to view the hospital resources for urban (and rural) blacks as part of the same health issue—the nation's hospital shortage—emphasized at this time by leading white liberal political and welfare reformists. This consonance between black medical leaders and national medical reformism was largely the result of two developments. First, blacks had participated strongly in both the military and domestic mobilization for World War II. Thus, black social and political leaders intensified their claims for federally regulated mechanisms to ensure full equality for blacks in all aspects of national life. To Rayford W. Logan, the prominent Howard University scholar, the overriding concern of black American leadership throughout World War

II was equal national participation. Writing in a 1944 collection of essays by some of the nation's leading blacks, *What the Negro Wants*, Logan identified six "irreducible fundamentals of first-class citizenship for all Negroes": equality of opportunity; equal wages for equal work; equal protection of the laws; equality in voting; abolition of segregation in public accommodations; and respect for the human dignity of black Americans.[36]

Mary McLeod Bethune, black America's most esteemed female educational leader, enunciated similar claims in her commentary "Certain Inalienable Rights." Bethune stressed the commonality between America's international war against dictatorship, and black American's struggle at home for civil rights and an end to lynchings. Other national objectives for blacks she stressed included voting rights, equal access to employment opportunities, and expansion of federal programs in public housing, social security, health, education, and welfare relief.[37] The nation's black medical leadership, then, reflected a rising black collective self-awareness and political idealism.

Second, in addition to the general rise in black political assertiveness nationally, black medical and social welfare leadership was becoming even more wedded to the relationalist paradigm: the construction of specific health problems of the black city communities as interconnected with a web of social and economic deprivations. The relationist paradigm was not simply a "political" viewing of black–white disease mortality and morbidity discrepancies. It led the black medical professional and research community down a unique path of sociomedical consciousness and policy activism in the fight to control infectious (and later, chronic and behavioral) disease among blacks.

The black relationist paradigm diverged with traditional medical and sociological multifactorialism on three levels: the development of medical knowledge, epidemiological knowledge, and sociological critique. Theoretically the central purpose of medical knowledge is to identify causation. But initially, according to TB historian J. G. Scadding, medical practitioners can "go no further than description of a recognizable combination of symptoms and signs," yielding a working, clinical description for diagnosing patients with this particular syndrome. The typical route for modern medical research has been to delve (often for periods of years, decades, or longer) deeper into the organ and substrate to get at even more precise abnormalities or pathogenesis in organs, physiological systems, even genetic systems. Even when this advance to identify microbiological causation reach plateaus, clinicians still have available a more sophisticated basis for categorizing patients with "a disease."[38] By contrast, the black medical practitioner, absorbed in the relationist paradigm, was committed to mastering as well as *applying* the latest clinical description of a disease. At those points when medicine's pursuit of substrate causation through clinical research became befuddled, relationists tended to look "outward" to the social realm at such forces as racism or poverty for the "causes" of the disease's prevalence as clinically defined in its present state. They approached medical care policy on this premise as well.

After World War II the Hill-Burton hospital construction program accelerated hospital growth. Thus, the nation's health care establishment had at its core a huge (federal) government-medical nexus geared to support traditional multifactorial paradigms. The Public Health Service's anti-VD programs during the 1930s was a prototypical outgrowth of this nexus. The central aim of this medical establishment's health care policy was clinical detection and curative treatment. But black relationists were concerned more with identifying and reducing the social forces in the black community that they believed tended to produce the excess black disease mortality and morbidity rates. Conversely, black medical relationalism considered unreasonable the notion or faith that progress, even revolutions, in clinical medicine and chemotherapy automatically resulted in broad social benefits. True, medical (clinical) innovations could be extremely effective in eliminating or managing a disease (or, as in the case of genetic disease, protecting offspring) in the individual. But to black medical leadership there was no guarantee these new cures would wind their way democratically into all segments of society at large, including blacks living in poverty or segregation, and reduce the black American's disproportionate suffering or mortality.[39]

In their assessment of the causes for higher mortality rates for urban black poor, the black medical community did not view deaths from communicable or degenerative diseases as etiologically disjointed. Instead, they approached these diseases as one common threat to black community health. Indeed, what is most fascinating for our purposes, as we view the post–World War II social and medical response to mass illness of black Americans on both sides of the nation's racial divide, is that the growth in scientific medical innovations during and immediately following World War II was paralleled by an intensification of the idea among black American medical and community health leaders that mass diseases of blacks were social and economic in origin.

Articulating the subtleties of the relationist paradigm was the wrenching burden that black medical leadership had to bear as they tried to win medical and political support for their health policies. Black relationists had to assert their common, historically and socially determined "racial" unity—traditionally used by their racial community in its political and legal struggle for equality—to advance their emphasis on *nonracial* causes for higher black mortality and morbidity patterns, and expose the myopia of medical perceptions that these sickness patterns were genetically unique to members of the black "race." Paul Cornely took on this task in his publications in professional and lay periodicals. In 1945 he wrote an article on black public health issues for the Urban League, "Health Assets and Liabilities of the Negro." As he summarized the seriousness of TB, venereal disease, and infant mortality among black Americans, Cornely warned that "the reader must not infer that there is such an entity as a 'Negro Health Problem,' for the health achievements and problems of this racial group are merely expressions of the total health situation of the country."[40]

A precise reading of black medical leadership's relational idea-system was given by W. Montague Cobb, the Howard University medical school professor, in an essay he wrote in 1946 for an academic audience. At this time Cobb was a leading force behind the NAACP's National Medical Committee, the members of which saw themselves as voicing the national health aspirations of black America. They agitated firmly for the NAACP's health program because, as Cobb stated shortly after World War II, the Association was "the oldest, largest and most representative organization of the fourteen million [black] American citizens who constitute the nation's largest minority."[41] He assessed the effort to lower the black–white mortality differential as requiring not a deemphasis on clinical research and specialization, but rather a broader application of what these new knowledge fields had revealed to date. Cobb was thrilled by the revolution in modern medical knowledge that his profession was witnessing:

Today the agents responsible for nearly every disease due to micro-organisms have been identifed and effective treatments developed. With the x-ray and its aids, most of the vital internal organs can be visualized. Great advancement has been made in the understanding of live processes and their derangement. Laboratory techniques can indicate the efficiency with which most organ systems function and the kinds of damage they suffer. Against infections the sulfa drugs, penicillin and other antibiotics are powerful weapons. . . . The development of specific vaccines and antisera has made it possible to stamp out certain diseases, like smallpox, and to minimize the effects of others, like whooping cough and measles. Antisepsis and fluid therapy, including blood and blood substitutes, have reduced the risks of major surgery and of accidental shock when promptly treated.[42]

Cobb and the other NAACP Medical Committee members also believed that America's distribution of medicine for the military during World War II had netted stupendous results. "In the emergency of the War there was a magnificent demonstration that we knew how to coordinate and organize all our vast medical knowledge and resources to make available to each member of the armed forces the kind of medical attention he needed." Yet, with the military conflict now terminated, this medical knowledge explosion had not flourished into a system of distribution of care adequate for blacks because of segregation or lack of financial resources. The peacetime nation has "allowed our social machinery for distributing medical care to fall lamentably behind advances in medical science," Cobb wrote. Among the nation's medical authorities, "[w]e have more or less indifferently permitted the survival of a system which dealt with health as a purchasable commodity and operated to the effect that one was entitled only to such medical care as he could pay for."[43]

Black medical leaders did not place highest priority on integration of hospitals and health centers. During these years before *Brown v. Board of Education in Topeka,* to many black medical professionals widescale integration seemed a futile pursuit especially in the South. Instead, their emphasis was on national health insurance, essentially an economic reform measure. They believed this universal repayment plan would open the accessibility to services for all of the nation's needy regardless of race or income, and at the same time finance the black physician and black hospital network. Cobb represented the NAACP's National Medical Committee at the hearings for the Wagner–Murray–Dingell (S. 1606) national health program bill in April 1946. This bill, a modified, angrily debated version of Senator Robert F. Wagner's comprehensive health insurance bill that had foundered in 1939, would give health insurance to all Americans paying Social Security taxes and their families.[44] Cobb stressed "the NAACP regards S. 1606 as one of the most progressive and potentially beneficial pieces of legislation of recent years [and] acutely needed by our 14,000,000 American Negro citizens." He criticized the American Medical Association's (AMA) counterproposal for "voluntary prepayment plans" as useless "to the poorly circumstanced of the American population of whom Negroes constitute the largest group." Because of their high premiums, private or voluntary health coverage plans simply were not available to low-income Americans "so that still the people who need medical care most are not able to provide for it."[45]

The National Medical Committee doctors and other leading black physicians harbored intense disfavor toward the AMA which at this time continued to sanction the racial exclusion of black doctors by its local or county medical societies throughout many regions of the country.[46] Thus, it is not surprising that the Committee emphasized it "would be unequivocally and unalterably opposed" to the administration of the proposed national health insurance plan through the AMA or local white-controlled medical societies. The plan, according to Cobb, would have to "be entirely in the hands of responsible public officials."[47]

E. I. Robinson and the NMA also advocated S. 1606. Robinson told Congress's Committee on Education and Labor at a 1946 hearing on the bill that the NMA appreciated the democratic character of this measure. Its adoption would further the general welfare clause in the Constitution "whereby the Federal Government assumes the responsibility to see to it that the welfare of every individual in the Nation will be adaquately safeguarded." Furthermore, Robinson emphasized that the great gap in the health status of the nation's blacks and whites was rooted in economics: "The health problems of the Negro are inextricably tied up with his economic situation rather than with any inherent racial factor." Because millions of blacks lacked the income to "purchase health," Robinson urged that the passage of S. 1606 was of "particular importance."[48]

As mentioned earlier, organized medicine's battle against Senator Wagner's original national health insurance bill had triumphed during the 1930s. The mainstream medical profession's opposition to the Wagner–Murray–Dingell bill was equally aggressive, and by 1949 essentially destroyed its legislative viability.[49] This political reality reinforced the relationist medical paradigm of the nation's black health leaders, causing them to fundamentally shift their collective health policy objectives. Their efforts became increasingly aimed at improving the flow of medical care to black urban (and poor rural) populations. The functional scope and supply of these new resources—hospital beds, and health centers and districts—would be coordinated by government agencies. In short, black medical leadership wanted to get blacks suffering from disease into the proper medical setting regardless of the financial (or consumer) status of these medically needy blacks. Months after the Committee on Education and Labor hearings on S. 1606, Midian Bousfield asserted that this approach was the most feasible path for future efforts to reduce excess black mortality.

Addressing the NMA's annual conference as chair of its Commission on Hospitals and Medical Education in Louisville, Kentucky, in 1946, Bousfield sketched the ideal health system for black Americans. He urged that optimal distribution of medical services could be provided by surrounding a chain of general hospitals with health centers along the lines of the approaches of New York City, which had a closely packed population, and Los Angeles County, a more loosely settled population center. The ideal health system should accommodate 50,000 to 200,000. Bousfield argued that this health care model would provide for "the decentralization of public health administration and works best [for] a more or less homogenous neighborhood population." The health center network should entail both diagnostic and treatment clinics, have active programs in health education and preventive measures, and control both public and voluntary health agencies. Bousfield's "self-contained" health departments, then, would hinge neither on the racial integration of housing nor on black and white hospitals and physician communities. All such medical resources, although generally segregated, would be subordinated to the health center's coordinating network.[50]

Black medical and social welfare strategists immediately following World War II also emphasized producing and upgrading the supply of black physician-specialists. Absolute segregation of medical schools was becoming obsolete as early as the end of World War II. But both black and white medical activists assumed that housing and hospital segregation would essentially remain in place; moreover, both groups believed that optimal medical care was rendered through a physician-centered system. Therefore, another key feature of black medical leadership's health care plans stressed the need for the production of as many black physician-specialists as possible. These medical leaders, teaming up with white liberal medical educators and philanthropists, directed their energies toward dismantling institutionalized economic barriers that tended to restrict the education of greater numbers of blacks in the specialties.

The earliest and most successful of such interracial efforts was the National Medical Fellowships (NMF) organization centered in Chicago. Founded in 1946, the NMF was first designed to reconstruct the staff of Provident Hospital in Chicago, the nation's most famous black hospital, following the war. Funded primarily by both local and national white philanthropists, NMF quickly spread as a national conduit for promising black medical students and physicians interested in training in the specialty fields (education available almost exclusively at predominantly white academic medical institutions) or becoming medical school teachers or researchers. In addition to providing fellowships, scholarships, and loans for postgraduate training, NMF also assisted promising black candidates in identifying nonsegregated specialty-training programs.[51]

Integration of blacks into medical educational and public health institutions was by 1950 irreversible. Ironically, this meant that those black institutions traditionally most effective in stimulating community health projects throughout the nation's black population were merged into larger, predominantly white-controlled organizations. For example, following its takeover by the Public Health Service, the National Negro Health Week movement had been operated as this agency's Office of Negro Health Work. But in 1950 this office was discontinued and its functions replaced by the Special Programs Branch, a unit deeper inside the Public Health Service's organizational pyramid. Also, around this time the National Association of Colored Graduate Nurses disbanded and merged with the American Nurses' Association.[52]

3

During the 1950s, the relational paradigm gained more momentum among black medical and social welfare strategists, not coincidentally at this time when the AMA was continuing to battle for defeat of any legislation that would increase the supply of physicians or medical care coverage for needy social sectors (black or white).[53] Increasingly the principal goal in health policy for the National Urban League and the NAACP became obtaining a medical setting for all needy black citizens by exposing and politically forcing hospitals to remove racial barriers. During 1954 the Urban League informed President Eisenhower that black American health lagged because they were "literally at the bottom of the pile" not only in income, living conditions, and educational level, but also for receiving "adequate facilities for hospitalization and medical care." Having conducted surveys on health problems of blacks and hospital discrimination in several major cities, the Urban League stressed that these social and medical conditions were interlinked and had to be addressed simultaneously.[54]

The health care plans proposed by Charles S. Johnson during

the mid-1950s also exemplified the shift in the policy orientation of black medical strategists away from struggle for the "universal benefits" of national health insurance toward a pragmatic, coordinated network of medical services within black urban and rural communities. A longtime head of research for the National Urban League and Fisk University scholar, Johnson was one of the few black sociologists at this time respected nationally outside of traditional black academic and social policy circles. His view represented a new emphasis, not on the issue of financial access to medical care for all Americans, but on specifying what organizational network of medical care resources would most immediately reduce black community health problems.

Two speeches by Charles S. Johnson on health delivered in 1954 indicate clearly that he and other black medical and social welfare leaders (1) interpreted "relationally" the roots of specific health problems of blacks, whether these problems were communicable, deficiency, or chronic diseases; and (2) declared the need for new, broad-ranging medical services for black communties to intervene in this environmentally produced, multidisease cycle. Citing the slum living conditions of blacks (both in the central cities and rural regions) as well as the overbearing power of folk health practices throughout black communities, Johnson stressed that black health "is not only a community problem and a community responsibility but a national problem and a national responsibility." He pressed the federal government both to surmount southern white political opposition toward placing federal funds in the hands of needy black populations, and to spend more on health coverage plans, such as the Wagner Maternal and Child Health bill: "The fact that many southern Congressmen, more concerned with preventing Federal interference with a cherished social pattern than with the needs of their constituents, oppose this legislation, confuses the issue, but does not lessen the responsibility."[55]

Johnson stressed four measures that would alleviate black medical-service needs. First, he favored expansion of group-specialty practices in which small, but diverse numbers of specialists housed their services together or, at least, tightly organized referral arrangements with general practitioners. Group practice had the benefit of bringing specialists trained in the latest advances in diagnosis and clinical therapy to the average patient.[56] "The tremendous increase of medical knowledge, particularly in the specialized fields, has made it impossible for one individual to encompass all of it," he remarked. Thus, the group practice made a variety of specialties available to a patient while encouraging coordinated medical record-keeping and surveillance. It also was an arrangement that did not challenge residential segregation because it facilitated black general practitioners and specialists working together in all-black communities.

Second, as Bousfield had some years earlier, Johnson stressed "regionalism" to interconnect health services. Group practices, hospitals, and health departments could come together under one organizing body or health service district to ensure efficient screening, diagnosis, and treatment services for the entire range of a large population's health problems. Third, Johnson emphasized the need to educate black families to understand the benefits of modern medical care and the importance in putting aside folk health ways for physician and hospital care.[57]

Finally, Johnson believed that mixed arrangements for financing the purchase of medical services was the most feasible approach for providing economic assess to health services. He enumerated the growth of both government funds for health care as well as voluntary medical financing programs. The rise in federal revenues for state and local public health had stimulated state and local expenditures for public health to increase from $36 million in 1935 to about $152 million annually by 1948. From 1920 to 1950 the number of local health departments increased from 131 to 1,734. While Johnson was encouraged by the rapid growth of voluntary prepayment health plans (exemplified by Blue Cross) and the growth in government spending on public health care, there was still the matter of medical services for those populations who were too poor to participate in any prepayment health insurance. These included families on public relief, many of the nation's elderly, and others with marginal incomes such as seasonal workers. For these groups, Johnson looked to additional government subsidies as the means to finance their medical care. "[G]overnment must take on a greater measure of responsibility for personal health services for low-income groups, and must continue and expand its support of the long-term institutional care of those suffering from mental disease, tuberculosis, or other chronic illness."[58]

During the mid- and latter 1950s, black health and civil rights activists in several major cities conducted local surveys to identify discrimination against blacks both in training and employment of black medical professionals, as well as admission and treatment of black community residents. This local activism was another shift away from pursuing the goal of universal access to medical care. Instead, these professionals attempted to galvanize black communities against local patterns of social and medical discrimination. It also subsumed concerns for TB and venereal diseases within these larger claims for more hospital services, black physicians, and financial assistance to pay for medical services.

During 1954 to 1956 the Detroit Commission on Community Relations convened the Medical and Hospital Study Committee to conduct a comprehensive survey of Detroit's black community and local medical institutions. The Committee, composed of local ministers, physicians, and civil rights leaders, investigated black admission policies at local medical schools, nurses' training programs at colleges and hospitals, medical staff appointments, and hospital bed utilization throughout the city's 47 general hospitals. The assumptions underlying the Medical and Hospital Study Committee's work was that the health care differential, and not a black–white mortality discrepancy due to a specific disease, had to be eliminated to equalize black and white health. The Committee's original charge was to study and document "facts relative to differentials in opportunities for training and practice, or in facilities and services available to minority groups, particularly Negroes." After the data was assembled, the Commission planned to pressure the faulty medical bodies to exercise "a single, high, non-racial standard of medical services to the Community."[59]

The Detroit Medical Study Committee found that only small numbers of blacks were attending the medical and nurses' education programs throughout local institutions. Also, while patient admissions were generally integrated, hospital distribution and bed assignments were fundamentally segregated.[60] The Committee pointed to de facto segregation as the major obstacle to equality in the local medical professional community and hospital distribution. It cited "two major factors involved in achieving this goal of nonracial utilization of bed facilities in the community's tax supported (governmental) and tax exempt (voluntary) hospitals. . . . The first relates to the racially representative character of the medical staff which is serving the hospital, and the second relates to the provision of bed facilities within the hospital without regard to race."[61] The Committee clearly perceived race, not class, as the major barrier to equitable health care for black Detroit. "Racial segregation has no place in present day community hospital operation," its report concluded. "The Negro citizen is legally, morally, and financially entitled to equal accommodation and use of hospital facilities, despite custom, practice, or formerly expedient patterns of service."[62] Similar local investigations excoriating racial discrimination in medical care fields and services occurred in Philadelphia, Chicago, and other major cities.[63]

4

A closer look at disease and race issues within the dominant health care sector during the 1950s and early 1960s reveals an important paradox. On the one hand, the leaders of black medical institutions and community groups were struggling to increase the awareness of the grinding health care needs within America's black community. On the other hand, the general medical research and public health establishment was methodically precluding any construction of a "black community health crisis." During the 1950s and early 1960s, most published medical discourse on TB and venereal disease, epidemiological surveys of these diseases, and policy making debates about eliminating these ailments referred to black populations (literally) as "nonwhites." This common practice of not using the identifier "Negroes" or "American blacks," but a term or what I call a "race-sign" ("nonwhite") denoting a vague, colored mass, served a number of interlocking functions within the medical and public health sectors, and American society generally.

First, the "white/nonwhite" approach subtly sustained the "scientific" functionality of the erroneous racialist conceptualization that disease susceptibility was primarily genetic in origin. Second, the practice reinforced the cultural and social psychological inferiorization of Afro-Americans, or what black cultural critics and sociologists like Ralph Elison and St. Claire Drake then called the Negro's "invisibility" and "self-identification problems."[64] Third, and most significant for this medical-social study, the white/nonwhite approach in epidemiological data and medical care policy reinforced epidemiological denial within the dominant health care segments (and the public and political sectors they strongly influenced) of the black community's ongoing crisis with TB and venereal disease. Chemotherapeutic innovations, natural immunization processes, and higher standards of living were indeed reducing general rates of TB and syphilis. But the mainstream medical sector's practice of disgarding the cultural and community identity of black victims of these diseases, while at the same time emphasizing the probability that a Negro or nonwhite racial factor was causally associated with higher susceptibility to these diseases, distanced this sector even farther from the black health paradigm developing within the black medical and health rights community.[65]

The general medical profession's disinterest in mounting a broad-scale effort to reduce TB and venereal disease striking heavily black communities was reinforced by several other developments. Optimism and apathy pervaded American public health leadership during the 1950s and early 1960s. The steep decline in TB mortality during the middle third of the twentieth century is one of the great achievements in American medical scientific and public health history. In 1932 TB had been responsible for about 79,000 deaths in the United States, or roughly one death per 1,600 population. Yet by 1952 TB deaths dropped to approximately 25,000; and 9,500 in 1962, or just 1 per 20,000 persons. In 1962 the black TB death rate was 11.5 per 100,000, nearly three times the white rate for that year, 4.2. This was still, of course, an immense decline from the TB death rates of blacks early in this century. In Manhattan, for example, from 1910 to 1950 TB mortality rates for blacks (nonwhites) dropped from 446 per 100,000 to 62 per 100,000.[66] This remarkable drop in TB mortality resulted from a combination of social and medical factors, most notably, the rise in sanitation, housing and food conditions, coupled with the wide dissemination of two much-heralded drugs, isoniazid and streptomycin, beginning in the early 1950s.[67]

The structural impact of the general reduction in TB on post-1950 American medical care was immense. A group of TB-specialists for the Public Health Service observed in 1956 that "[w]ith the advent of the new antituberculosis drugs, the need for prolonged stay in hospitals has been diminished, and care of tuberculosis patients at home has become increasingly accepted."[68] Overall, the number of beds allotted for TB patients dropped from 106,502 in 1951 to 12,401 by 1971. City-by-city health and political authorities closed down TB treatment facilities once needed for isolating and hospitalizing tuberculars for months or years. Between 1957 and 1962 the 20 public hospitals in New York for TB dropped to 12.[69]

A similar giant stride was made in venereal disease control immediately following World War II. In 1943 penicillin therapy was initiated, and a few years later, synthesized and applied on a mass scale. This new treatment could be applied in ambulatory or outpatient settings; it thus eliminated most hospitalization, which, in turn, greatly lowered the cost of medical care. There was a marked reduction in the cumulative after-effects of syphilis. In 1937 the mortality rate due to syphilis was 12 per 100,000, but by 1959 fell to 1.7 per 100,000. Similar dramatic declines in paresis and infant mortality due to syphilis occurred during this same period.[70]

These new pharmaceutical (curative) assaults on venereal disease and TB, moreover, reinforced faith in the traditional, multifactorial epidemic paradigm. By the late 1950s many in the medical community, public media, and lay community believed that the new chemotherapies had "solved" the TB and venereal disease problems. Researchers and health officials shifted their focus to clinical or family epidemiology. Public health work relating to TB and venereal disease concentrated on uncovering cases. In the area of TB control, the national health authorities centered on "intensive public health supervision" of nonhospitalized TB patients who could spread infections if they prematurely terminated treatment.[71] Some local political bodies such as those of New York City, Los Angeles County, Seattle, Milwaukee, Columbus, and Philadelphia, as well as California State even enacted laws allowing forcible hospitalization of "recalcitrant [TB] patients."[72]

At the national meetings of public health officials and TB experts, this optimistic and narrow concept of public health, which focused on the patient and not groups at risk or conditions and social behaviors that created this risk, prevailed. Moreover, there was no reference to mobilizing against the threat and effect of these diseases inside black communities. For example, in 1958 some 3,000 physicians, public health workers, and nurses gathered at the annual joint conference of the NTA and National Conference of Tuberculosis Workers. Leaders of the conference expressed some concern over the widening public and political apathy toward TB control measures. But these same conference leaders focused almost exclusively on medical therapeutic aspects of TB and related lung and cardiovascular diseases. Session topics focused on "drug therapy and hospitalization," "surgical treatment," "mimics of TB" (or atypical mycobacteria), "other chest diseases," "lung cancer," "natural resistance and therapy," and "protective measures." As for future directions, the prominent pathologist Esmond Long discussed natural susceptibility and the need to pursue "the unexpressed thought . . . that the characteristics [of natural resistance] are genetically linked with other [largely anatomical] factors that are truly pertinent to native resistence."[73]

In the South segregationists attempted to turn blacks' excessive TB mortality rates into justification for keeping white and black youths from attending integrated schools. These southerners cited data that showed black TB mortality was roughly four times greater than whites', and that the incidence rates of active cases among blacks exceeded whites by three times. According to Thomas F. Pettigrew, a leading sociologists of this period, "[s]egregationists . . . employ these data to argue that biracial schools in the South present a health hazard."[74]

5

As most American medical care institutions drifted into serving primarily those social segments that could afford hospital care (due to private, employment-related, or welfare-state health plans), the health problems facing black Americans not in these segments remained largely obscured. This medical care gap spurred even more militancy from black community medical and social activists. By the end of the 1950s and into the early 1960s momentum swelled greatly to make hospital integration the principal goal for black Americans' health care. Beginning in 1957 the NMA, the NAACP, the National Urban League, and the Medico-Chirurgical Society of the District of Columbia (the local black medical assocation) began coordinating what would become a series of seven yearly "Imhotep" conferences on integration of hospitals. These national meetings stressed three goals: legal measures to prohibit segregation in hospital services; termination of public funds for segregated hospital construction or maintenance; and direct negotiations with hospital adminstators and associations to encourage integrated hospital policies.[75]

The Imhotep conferences, virtually all of which were composed of black physicians and black hospital administrators, brought greater public visibility to black American medical leaders' opposition to segregated medical facilities. But the mainstream government and hospital establishment merely ignored this forum, in effect, segregating the Imhotep group from the most influential policy-making spheres for the nation's medical care. As Herbert Morais wrote a few years after the last (1963) Imhotep conference, the "effectiveness of these meetings was vitiated by the refusal of such powerful oganizations as the AMA, the American Hospital Association and various Protestant and Catholic hospital bodies to participate officially and actively in the [Imhotep] deliberations."[76]

During the early and mid-1960s, black American medical leaders shifted their health policy objectives toward mobilizing black community and interracial civil rights groups for direct action campaigns to force the integration issue. This new sociopolitical thrust for a total ban of racially discriminatory policies and practices in medical services, and professional education, and employment was sharply evident in the internal debate within the black medical community. Leaders of the NMA, as well as new clusters of urban black medical professionals and the black nursing community, voiced a common notion that united black community action was the most potent weapon to eliminate racial barriers in health care. This assertive black medical leadership believed that only confrontational civil-rights politics would in the end win black America's fight against the social diseases of poverty and racism, as well as the bodily diseases caused by infections and physical and mental debility.

A keynote address to the House of Delegates at the NMA's meeting in 1962 delivered by Dr. W. T. Armstrong described "the waters of the world [as] . . . troubled." Black America's dissatisfaction with discrimination was reaching a peak, Armstrong emphasized. "There is unrest . . . and the clamor of millions of people for equal opportunity and the right to be treated as human beings and as Americans, [which] brings into sharp focus the responsibility of the membership of the National Medical Association." He cited the many lawsuits in federal courts throughout the country aimed at prohibiting hospital segregation and amending the Hill–Burton Act to bar federal funds to disciminatory medical facilities. Most vexing, however, was the situation in the urban North. There, the status of blacks in medicine and health care was not simply a question of eliminating legalized racial barriers in medical schools or hospitals. Instead, blacks in the northern cities faced "the cumulative impact of poverty and ignorance at home, degraded neighborhoods, poor educational facilities, limited job opportunities and the ever-present fear of rebuttal."[77]

At this 1963 conference the NMA passed its stirring "Resolution in Support of Mass Protests Against Racial Discrimination." This measure permitted members to participate in protest activities under the official name of NMA with the approval of the president and board representative. It was in response to the militant initiatives of the NMA's president, John A. Kenney, Jr., who communicated to the membership that the first objective of his administration was the "continued fight against discrimination and segregation in medicine, in all forms." Kenney had urged passage of this resolution because "the temper of the times, the image of our organization, the dignity of our profession, and the obligations to our collective conscience, demand that we forthrightly declare the position of this body on the current [racial] revolution, lest most of us stand in violation of its law."[78]

During the early and mid-1960s the NMA worked at several levels to address the medical care needs of urban blacks. First, the association expanded its political and financial support for national civil rights organizations, especially the NAACP, but also CORE, SCLC, and SNCC. It also became one of the earliest and most vigorous lobbyists for Medicare.[79] Finally, the NMA encouraged political activism throughout the black physician community by mobilizing them to function as a pressure group on Congress and the president on civil rights issues. The NMA also provided clusters of doctors as medical workers for independent mass health rights movements such as the Medical Committee for Human Rights (MCHR).

During the summer of 1964 civil rights organizations in Mississippi put out an urgent request for a "medical presence" in that state, calling attention to the recent murders of James Chaney, Andrew Goodman, and Michael Schwerner. Scores of white and black health professionals based primarily in the North responded, organized into the MCHR, and journeyed south to work with local black medical professionals and community workers. By the spring of 1965 MCHR had branch groups in eight major cities, and such prominent sponsors as Paul Cornely, Benjamin Spock, Leslie Falk, and Walsh McDermott.[80] Dr. Aaron O. Wells, the national chairman of MCHR, wrote pridefully in a promotional letter issued March of 1965:

> Since [MCHR] was formed, our organization has continued to work and grow, as physicians, nurses, dentists, psychologists, medical students and other health professionals throughout the Nation have welcomed the opportunity to use their speicific health skills for the cause of Civil Rights. . . . We need no more dramatic reminder of the role we can play than was offered by Selma, Alabama. On that bloody Sunday afternoon, MCHR was there with 5 doctors, 4 nurses and our Mobile Health Unit to cooperate with local MD's.[81]

The MCHR eventually developed local groups in over thirty cities, including all of the major northern ones. Its major activity in these communities involved recruiting volunteers for medical and community support work in southern states. But MCHR became a organizational tool to fight inadequacies in health care communities of these northern cities as well. As one MCHR organizer emphasized, health and political conditions in northern cities were as much in need of MCHR support as were southern black communities:

> Of paramount importance to our contribution will be the effectiveness with which we apply medical presence in the Northern ghetto struggle. Certainly our support here must be strengthened and extended. In a sense, we can follow many of the precedents already established in the South by closely aligning ourselves with civil rights and local community civil groups in long-term presence of highlighting and exposing the insidious

and subtle discriminatory patterns that exist in the Northern health area.[82]

MCHR workers were eventually involved in setting up health programs for children living in impoverished neighborhoods, protest marches to integrate local hospitals, and programs to attract black and Hispanic youth to medical occupations.

By 1966 the approaches of black medical leadership to health care for black central city communities focused on developing flexible, decentralized means to deliver medical services at the neighborhood level. As had occurred in earlier periods of the century, an institutional bridge or superstructure developed between black medical and community welfare activism, on the one hand, and the mainstream medical establishment, on the other. In the 1920s municipalities and urban academic-medical centers employed the black public health sector as their initial vehicle to fight the black health crisis. During the 1930s and 1940s national voluntary health organizations and the federal government had utilized and incorporated black advisers, the National Negro Health Week program, and local black community health leaders.

But in the 1960s and early 1970s the modern "first line of defense" for the medical establishment and black community health activists was the resurrected comprehensive-care neighborhood health centers. Both black health care leadership and medical reformers spearheaded the drive to open such facilities with grants from the Office of Economic Opportunity (OEO). These OEO health care funds derived from the Economic Opportunity Act, which modern health care historians call "the single largest government-attack on poverty in American history."[83] The central requirement for such funds was that a grantee represent a local community institution interested in designing and operating a comprehensive health service facility—a facility based on plans "derived from the needs of the people to be served." Between 1965 and 1969 OEO made 104 comprehensive health services grants for such projects, most of which were administered by community hospitals (23 percent), medical schools (19 percent), health corporations (17 percent), health departments (13 percent), and OEO community action agencies and other nonprofit bodies (20 percent). Only a miniscule proportion of OEO projects were operated by medical societies (2 percent) or group practices (6 percent).[84]

But as the OEO community-based projects began to age, activist black-communtity health workers and reform-minded medi-

cal planners recognized that the OEO neighborhood health center
movement had fundamental, indeed fatal weaknesses. OEO-spon-
sored health programs were ill-defined superstructures with ambiva-
lent, often poorly focused constituencies. According to recent analysts of the programs, most OEO planners and field staff were
professionals who worked from their own abstract blueprints of target communties "rather than involving the poor themselves in strate-
gy design."[85] These blueprints neglected the shifting social structure
and community life of the central city black community. As Hatch
and Eng pointed out, "OEO programs were often planned as if poor
communities had no viable social organization or structure. They,
therefore, sought to create or sanction new structures rather than to
conduct a hard analysis of what existed."[86]

Effective or not, under the Nixon adminstration OEO's days
were numbered; in 1974 it was abolished by Congress. Afterwards,
the confusing array of medical care institutions and financial barriers
preventing uniform access to treatment services hurt most directly
America's poor. Most damaging was the scarcity of preventive health
services for mothers, infants, and youth; as well as the inadequate
mixture of medical services for the adult working and nonworking
populations due to their financial or geographic handicaps. The
view among most health care reformers at this time was that the
United States "has a nonsystem of medical care, no national health
goals, and only a series of competing short-range programs."[87]

Although the post–World War II period is seen generally by
contemporary historians as a high point in the integration of American medical care, actually black medical care leaders had experienced a growing isolation from the national medical and health policy agenda. This isolation also tended to reinforce these leaders'
outlook on the origins and extent of mass illness and diseases most
frequently prevalent among urban blacks, an outlook incompatible
with that of general organized medicine. As the relational paradigm
intensified among black American medical leaders, their policy focus
shifted. Pursuit of lowering the black–white mortality differential, to
them, became not the struggle for national health insurance for all
Americans, but for specific medical resources, no matter how funded, most needed by the central-city community.

Black health activists of the civil rights period concentrated
especially on forming a united civil rights–medical rights movement.
This health-rights movement strove to eliminate segregation in medical facilities; to open more training and employment opportunities at
these institutions for black doctors, nurses, and allied health work-

ers; and to build a network of community-based health services for the inner-city (and rural) poor. During the Nixon years, however, integration was removed from the agendas of the federal government and national media. The functional ties between the federally subsidized health care agencies, the black health care professional sectors, and impoverished black community segments with its health activists, were in effect dismantled. Both the mainstream medical care sector as well as health care institutions located in black neighborhoods stood ill-prepared to mount a broad campaign against the coming AIDS peril.

Chapter 6

Health Care Delivery and a People Divided: Facing the AIDS Epidemic

During the early 1980s, acquired immune deficiency syndrome (AIDS) became a national and worldwide public health issue. Within a few years the concentration of AIDS cases in the United States began to shift from mostly white male homosexuals to urban blacks and Hispanics. On the quantitative scale, AIDS in the black American population seems negligible compared to the TB scourge at the beginning of this century. In 1910 and 1920 black mortality from TB was estimated to be 446 per 100,000 and 263 per 100,00 respectively. These death rates tower over even the incidence rates of AIDS cases for blacks and Hispanics which were as of 1988, 34.9 per 100,000 and 28.9 per 100,000 respectively.[1] However, the dissimilar course of the AIDS outbreak throughout specific segments of the black and white American populations, as well as the emergent epidemic paradigms bear strong similarities to the communicable disease epidemics described earlier.

As the AIDS crisis gained media and political attention throughout America, the construction of a possible African racial connection to greater susceptibility for AIDS emerged throughout the nation's medical science and health care–sociology sectors. This sociomedical response paralleled that of the dominant medical and social welfare institutions confronting TB and syphilis epidemics earlier this century. The nation's health care system could not break from traditional and modern racialist discourse and institutional health care policy during the AIDS crisis. Thus, the health care and civic community leadership for much of the nation's black population was not significantly incorporated into the national health care establishment's AIDS programs. As of the late 1980s these programs made no substantial dent in controlling the spread of AIDS throughout the black and Hispanic American community.

1

Poor housing and sanitation were the environments that allowed TB to ravage black neighborhoods decades ago. But now contaminated needles shared by clusters of intravenous (IV) drug users typical in many poor black and white communities were the hub for transmission of the HIV infection throughout black America. Like the earlier TB crises, both the prevalence of and mortality from AIDS became concentrated throughout diversified segments of the black population, including youth and children. Currently not only do blacks compose about one-fourth of the nation's AIDS cases; they are also experiencing higher female, infant, and adolescent AIDS rates; AIDS via IV-drug-use or heterosexual transmission from IV-drug-user partners; and increased clinical TB cases largely associated with HIV infections.[2] For example, black women make up 51 percent of the total reported cases of female AIDS, and most are of child-bearing age. When one considers the cumulative incidence of AIDS (number of cases per million population of a particular subpopulation) by race, the data reveals that black males are about two and one-half times more likely to contract AIDS than white males, while black women are twelve times more likely to get AIDS than white women.[3] The high prevalence of AIDS within the black female population indicates that heterosexual transmission of AIDS is most frequently occuring in the black populations; and in the future the number of black children with AIDS will expand.[4]

National data for 1987 on children with AIDS revealed that blacks already composed about 54 percent of children under 13 years of age at the time of diagnosis for AIDS, while the remaining 46 percent were Hispanic (about 24 percent) and white (22 percent). The incidence of AIDS for black children nationwide was about 15 times larger than among whites and 9 times larger for Hispanics.[5] And, as Surgeon General Koop stated that same year, "just to increase our sense of horror at what is happening in the black and Hispanic communities, we suspect that these cases are vastly underreported."[6]

Similar to prior TB and syphilis epidemics, AIDS rates for blacks have been highest in the major cities. A breakdown of AIDS cases in New York City conducted in 1987 showed that the cases of AIDS prior to 1985 compared to post-1985 were centering increasingly among the city's blacks and Hispanics. As of 1987 slightly over one-fourth of the 40,000 AIDS cases reported nationally occurred in New York City.[7] Before 1985 the proportion of white cases was 52 percent, but dropped to 44 percent by 1987, while the percentage of black cases grew from 27 to 32 percent.[8] By December 1987, AIDS analysts in New York City wrote in the *New England Journal of Medicine* that about 500,000 people in metropolitan New York City were believed to be infected with HIV. Blacks and Hispanics were becoming increasingly dominant in this population. According to the New York City researchers, "[a]t the outset, AIDS was considered primarily a disease of white homosexual or bisexual men. However, with time, AIDS has become increasingly frequent among intravenous drug abusers, particularly those who are black or Hispanic, among newborns of women positive for the human immunodeficiency virus (HIV), and to a lesser degree, among recipients of blood or blood products adminstered before March 1985."[9]

In hospitals that service large populations of inner-city, low-income blacks, the HIV infections rates have turned out to be exceedingly high. In Baltimore during 1987–88, Johns Hopkins Hospital studied blood samples of 2,302 emergency-room patients, about 75 percent of whom were black, and discovered 119 or 5.2 percent of all patients surveyed were infected with AIDS. The seroprevalence of HIV was 4.8 percent for black patients, 1.6 percent for whites. Black men between the ages of 30 to 34 had the highest age-specific seroprevalence rates (11.4 percent).[10] The predominantly black and Hispanic South Bronx section of New York City apparently has one of the highest AIDS rates in the world. Tests of blood samples of 143 emergency-room patients at one South Bronx hospital (Bronx-Lebanon Medical Center) revealed that 23 percent, aged from 13 to 92, were HIV positive. Sixty percent of the infections had been transmitted by IV-drug use, 20 percent by sex with drug users, but only 10 percent through homosexual activity and another 10 percent via exposure to both homosexual or drug-abuse activities. As New York City's health commissioner Stephen C. Joseph remarked, "This virus is concentrating geographically, targeting and focusing on the poor and areas of high drug use. We know we are seeing increased infection and disease rates."[11]

Studies derived from New York City's Health and Hospitals Corporation (HHC), the largest municipal hospital system in the United States, provided a demographic picture of AIDS prevalence markedly different from that of San Francisco where white-male homosexual cases dominated. The HHC is comprised of eleven acute care facilities, five neighborhood family care centers, five long-term care facilities, and the city's emergency care services. Most of San Francisco's AIDS patients (based on 1985 data) were white (88 percent) and homosexual (83 percent). By contrast the HHC's AIDS patients were largely IV-drug users (62 percent) as well as children (5 percent) and heterosexual sex partners (11 percent) of IV-drug users. One HHC researcher emphasized, "The HHC's AIDS patient population comes almost entirely from minority groups, black or Hispanic, which account for 89 percent of the caseload in HHC institutions."[12]

In Newark, where one-third of the residents exist below the poverty line and homelessness is among the nation's highest, AIDS has been striking wide clusters of black and Hispanic families. At the end of 1988, 83 percent of the city's 1,110 AIDS cases were black and 11 percent Hispanic. Since nearly four-fifths of the AIDS cases in Newark are linked to IV drug use, the incidence of heterosexual transmission far exceeds the national rate. According to a coordinator for the National Minority Outreach Initiative Grant Program for the Centers for Disease Control (CDC), "In cities like Newark, AIDS has became a disease of the family. We're talking about women, children, men. It's not skipping over anyone." [13] The wide demographic spectrum of black AIDS victims throughout urban America made the association of this disease with black people visible, for sharply different reasons, to both the mainstream health care and black communities.

2

There were roughly three stages in the responses of the medical community and national health agencies to the TB and syphilis epidemics during the first half of this century. First, a period occurred when racialist models generated by medical authorities became popular. The health researchers and officials relied on sketchy mortality and morbidity data, as well as personal impression and social stereotypes to maintain the idea that blacks were the more natural carriers of or the most susceptible sector to these infectious diseases. The second phase involved information-building in which data on the magnitude and etiology of the diseases was accumulated and multifactorial perspectives expanded, tending to counterbalance prior racialism. Third, there was a period in which epidemiological denial occurred or black public health workers (professional and lay activists) were recruited into a superstructure with primary duties in black communities not reached adequately by the dominant medical and public health status quo.

Compared to TB and syphilis, the current medical research community has made incredibly fast progress in establishing the microbiological workings of AIDS, its pathogenesis and modes of transmission. Thus, it would seem that unlike the earlier TB and syphilis periods, racialism would not be a factor in the sociomedical response to AIDS. However, two developments within the general medical and sociological communities's research and policy discourse on AIDS have sustained a strong racialist theme throughout the AIDS crisis: first, the rise of the thesis that AIDS originated in Africa, and, second, the frequent practice of employing racial (biogenetic) variables in explaining the higher AIDS rates for black Americans.

As AIDS initially became a national issue, the assertion circulated by many within the United States and Western medical and social science communities was that the disease emerged among Africans or Haitians. Consequently, the idea spread rapidly throughout the media and general public that AIDS had a black Haitian or African origin.[14] The thesis that an African factor underlied the origins and spread of AIDS was a corollary of the common practice in United States (and Western) biomedical and health care research of positing via race-signs or codes a biogenetic difference or deficiency in "blacks" as a primary variable behind black–white disease differentials.[15] As we emphasized earlier, throughout the post–World War II decades a synchronic, genotypical concept of race, different in its technical usage but not in its social meaning from the earlier diachronic (evolutionary) racialism, became a common fixture in medical and policy research. Officials of Haiti and African nations, as well as health workers and researchers with firsthand familiarity with health conditions in specific African locales, questioned vigorously the idea that AIDS emerged in Africa or that there has been some sort of African racial factor associated with the spread of AIDS. But these questions have only recently come to light.[16] In the meantime, subsurface racialism, through race-signs, remained a key linchpin in medical and social scientific explanations for the apparently higher AIDS prevalence in Africa and Haiti.

While first- and second-stage perceptions (based either on racialism or multifactorialism) of a racial susceptibility to AIDS ferment, the nation's medical and public health sectors have just recently entered the third stage, the creation of a black public health sector to work at the community level against the rapid spread of AIDS among blacks and Hispanics. The most prominent federal action has been the formation of the National Minority AIDS Council, supported by the National Institute of Mental Health. The Council has coordinated conferences and forums throughout many communities that have resulted in the development of coordinated local public awareness programs. The CDC has initiated a number of programs designed specifically to reach black or Hispanic populations. In 1987 the CDC operated 55 AIDS Health Education/Risk Reduction (HE/RR) Programs. Twenty-one (38 percent) were targeted for blacks and 15 (28 percent) for Hispanics. The CDC's program for prevention of perinatal AIDS is mainly for populations in New York City, northern New Jersey, and Miami. Minority organizations and public relations businesses (through subcontracts) started getting CDC funds to promote media campaigns more suitable for black and Hispanic language and communication patterns.[17]

As of the start of 1988, however, the CDC still had virtually no programs in place to address the IV-drug-abuse and sociobehaviorial aspects at the heart of the black communities' AIDS problem. Moreover, little research had been conducted on IV-drug users in relation to AIDS prevention programs. Nationwide, except for studies done in large cities on samples of addicts entering treatment programs, there was little data or information on patterns of needle-sharing in diverse drug-using populations, on addicts who inject amphetamines or cocaine, or heroin users that do not submit to treatment.[18] Data on HIV prevelance in or treatment options for black middle-class population remained nonexistent. Nor were there any substantial CDC programs to encourage voluntary testing so as to cut off transmissions by the estimated hundreds of thousands of asymptomatic carriers of HIV. The large-scale use of black community languages and media, community workers, and traditional cultural institutions were also generally lacking. Finally, the CDC minority initiatives had yet to combine AIDS programs for medically needy black populations with other health initiatives such as those concerned with lung cancer, adolesecent pregnancy, and family planning.[19]

Indeed, America's federal public health and medical establishment had by 1988 a long way to go nationally to catch up with other developed nations in the battle of AIDS. This is clear when one compares the sporadic community-based AIDS initiatives of the various cities and states having substantial populations of AIDS victims and HIV-risk groups, with Sweden's programs. In Sweden, government and community initiatives to fight HIV have been given priority and implemented at all three of the interlinked levels of prevention: tertiary, secondary, and primary.[20] The tertiary focus has been on the medical care of patients with AIDS. This has been provided in four settings: within a special infectious disease hospital or general hospital; home-care system staffed by largely lay persons; large-scale outpatient services; and home-based medical care. Hemophiliacs are treated in specialized clinics and also benefit from a voluntary organization. One feature of this Swedish clinical program is particularly impressive: there are built-in services to relieve the psychological trauma the HIV patients and their families face.[21]

Secondary and primary prevention pertains to detection of the disease as early as possible and the curtailment of its spread to individuals at risk. In Sweden to reduce the anxiety of voluntary STD testing there is a venereal disease law that requires the physician diagnosing HIV in a patient to arrange for the patient and his/her close kin to receive psychosocial support (provided free of charge by governmental funds). As for preventing infection, the Swedish approach considered both the HIV and the IV-drug abuse epidemics as intertwined. Once a substantial capacity of service for medical and psychological care of those tested for HIV had been established, the police and criminal justice system were recruited in the anti-HIV initiative to implement volunatry testing of drug addicts with whom they come into contact (almost none of the drug addicts refuse the HIV test).[22]

At the state level, programs to distribute culture-specific prevention information to blacks and other minorities did emerge by 1988, albeit in bits and pieces. In New York, California, Pennsylvania, Maryland, Delaware, North Carolinia, Ohio, Indiana, Michigan, and Illinois, state health offices have tried increasingly to disseminate information that would intensify AIDS awareness in black communities. Most of these states funneled their educational initiatives and materials through community-based AIDS organizations already operating in high-incidence urban areas. In Pennsylvania, private donations funded minority AIDS education programs through a large local community AIDS organization, the Philadelphia AIDS Task Force. The state of California, which in 1988 set aside one-fourth of its AIDS education budget for minority programs, funded a broadly based AIDS project in Los Angeles targeted for black gay and bisexual men.[23]

Finally, a number of states also funded specific medical care services for AIDS patients at hospitals that have large black patient populations. By 1987 New York State, for instance, was spending about 380 million dollars annually on the care and treatment of persons with AIDS. This annual sum is expected to increase to about 1 billion dollars in 1991. Overall, however, very few of the state initiatives tied into traditional black civic or folk community institutions. Maryland has been an exception to this pattern. Its statewide AIDS initiative is using a black community network that includes the NAACP, church and neighborhood groups, and the black media.[24]

Some municipal governments of major cities with substantial

black populations started AIDS programs designed for black and Hispanic residents. In 1985 the District of Columbia established an interagency task force on AIDS. Subsequently, the city council passed an
ordinance, the AIDS Health-Care Response Plan (1986). The measure
set aside over one million dollars annually for public education programs and support services for Persons With AIDS (PWAs) and their
families.[25] A somewhat similar local program has emerged in Newark
(N.J.). In 1988 a Task Force on AIDS was established by the city of
Newark composed of local elected officials, community leaders and
residents, medical workers, educators and scientists. Thus far, the
Task Force has held citywide conferences, distributed literature as
well as campaigned for home care of persons infected with HIV but
not yet in need of hospitalization. Other efforts included recruiting
ex-drug addicts for outreach work and developing homes for children with AIDS.[26]

3

Compared to earlier periods in the twentieth century when
infectious diseases posed epidemic threats, the black community's
collective response to the AIDS epidemic has been skewed, generating little pressure on national medical and public health authorities.
During the TB epidemic early in this century, we observed that public health voluntarism was widespread among black civic and church
groups, culminating in the Negro Health Week movement started in
1915. During the 1950s and 1960s, the medical and social battle
against mass illness stemming from ghettoization, rural poverty, and
violence against civil rights workers was led largely by black medical
professionals and allied white physicians and community health
activists. By contrast, the professional health care and welfare elements of America's current black community have not unified against
the AIDS threat. In New York City, for example, an analysis of community-based resources in place as of 1988 by the city's commissioner of health described a variety of efforts. Some services were geared
toward persons with AIDS, others toward the public generally, and
finally some toward at-risk populations. But no AIDS programs were
identified that were specifically operated by predominantly black
organizations or black HIV-risk populations of the city.[27]

There have been indications that traditional networks within
major black communities are beginning to meet the AIDS threat head
on. For example, black clergy of ten of New York City's largest black
churches began a united effort to deliver sermons about the growing

peril of AIDS to black residents. Overall they intended to mobilize some 600 black congregations.[28] In San Francisco, when Commissioner of Health Naomi Gray issued a challenge during 1986 to local black social leaders to explore the impact of AIDS on their community, she received an outpouring of interest. A permanent black communty-based organization was formed, the Black Coalition On AIDS. One of its workers described the birth of this organization:

> [Commissioner Gray] had seen spiraling funding for AIDS education and few activities directed toward the Black population. Her invitation was a challenge to the Balck community to define and advocate for our own needs. Out of that challenge we have created a broadly based organzation including over 200 individuals and agencies committed to the education and service needs of our community.

The coalition has focused on providing technical assistance and informational materials to social service agencies throughout the city's black communities on AIDS; promoted an AIDS Awareness Month program; and assisted in the design and implementation of one of the nation's first surveys on attitudes and behaviors in black communities germane to building more effective programs in AIDS prevention.[29]

Nonetheless, compared to the earlier black public health voluntarism to combat TB and venereal disease—such as the black community- and federally-subsidized National Health Week movement during the 1930s—organized efforts within the national lay black community to fight AIDS have been meager for several reasons. The black community faces behavioral, cultural, and demographic factors that make community-based mobilization against the spread of AIDS particularly difficult. Urban black communities not conducive to community-based AIDS initiatives often exhibit homophobia, widespread particularly in its large religious sector. Also, there is a general mistrust of government-operated programs that many poor blacks harbor due to perceived or experienced patterns of mistreatment or negligence at the hands of other (nonmedical) government agents (police, caseworkers, etc.).[30]

The behavioral characteristics of black adult subgroups most likely within the HIV-positive population are particularly resistant to collective mobilization against AIDS (or, for that matter, any other public health menace). In California, the great number and variety of community-based AIDS organization emerged "in response to the [largely] homogenous patient population (i.e., gay and bisexual males) in that state."[31] However, we have emphasized that the heaviest population infected with HIV in black communities are diversified, centering around IV-drug users and their sex-partners and offspring. Unlike the urban gay community, the IV-drug–user sector resists organization by black community or professional health workers if the workers themselves are "outsiders" to the IV-drug–user subculture. Furthermore, drug-treatment, medical care and social rehabilitation programs for lower-class drug users is one of the most neglected and disorganized sectors in the nation's human service network.[32] Donald R. Hopkins, former assistant surgeon general, has stated bluntly that "AIDS will not be controlled in black and Hispanic communities without more effective prevention of drug abuse and widespread access to treatment centers for drug abusers."[33]

There are gender and cultural characteristics of the black community's potential and actual AIDS population that also work to obstruct formal AIDS programs in black communities. I stressed previously that there is a high proportion of women and children in the HIV-risk black population, many of whom live in extreme poverty and who are illiterate. Like the IV-drug–user population, the impoverished female sector—black, Hispanic, and white spouse of a black—is but another segment in the black community that tends to have no influence in those local or national political sectors that control the planning and operations of local health care institutions. On the one hand, these female poor face virtually insurmountable daily living circumstances, and, on the other, they are faceless to the ingrown power of political and medical expert structures.[34]

Workers in black/Hispanic community-based AIDS programs in Newark and New York City offer case-histories of the difficulties these programs encounter. They usually find IV-drug users and their typically female-headed household networks trapped in overbearing economic circumstances. Frequently women advised to leave their IV-drug–user partners refuse adamantly because they will inevitably become homeless without their male partner's financial support. Other community residents shun any contact with "government" AIDS workers, while Hispanic residents (black and white) confront language barriers and cultural differences, as well as fear governmental reprisals for illegal immigration status. Last, Newark's and New York City's hard-core poor frequently refuse the HIV test because they would rather live with the uncertainty of AIDS than experience rejection by their sparse but meaningful world of kin and friends. At a Newark drug rehabilitation facility that provides AIDS services, one counselor commented:

All they [i.e., clients at the facility] have sometimes are their buddies. The don't want to be shut out. They've all heard the stories about people being kicked out of the projects because they were HIV-positive. Many didn't have anywhere to go but the streets.[35]

As for promoting the use of condoms by focusing on female sex-partners of IV-drug users, this too has often led to naught, given the powerless conditions poor, minority women at HIV risk typically encounter. One staff worker for the Foundation for Research on Sexually Transmitted Diseases in New York City described their situation bluntly:

if you are Hispanic and living in a barrio and you have very little food for your kids, and your guy comes home and you say, 'okay, now here is the condom for you to wear,' and in response he hits you across the face and walks out and you have no more food for the kids, then you do not say it again.[36]

Another complexity preventing the emergence of a coherent anti-AIDS movement thoughout the national black community has been the absence of a social movement comparable to the Civil Rights movement. The black political sector has been unable to "politicize" the need for more funds and resources to expand fundamentally standard and integrated AIDS programs for medically needy black populations. Unlike the black medical and social welfare activists during the immediate post–World War II period, the present black health care activism cannot link the AIDS issue with larger drives for black community betterment, civil justice, and economic power. A clearly defined and effective mass movement such as the grass-root voter-registration campaigns of the 1960s and 1970s simply did not emerge during the 1980s.

4

The national government and medical-welfare establishment have also failed to penetrate the sociological, attitudinal, behavioral, and gender complexities at the source of the AIDS epidemic throughout black America for two primary reasons. First, it has been uninterested in taking the lead to weld together a comprehensive network of black community-based health providers to focus on the AIDS emergency. Second, health care policymakers have not recognized that historically and culturally the approaches to health and sickness, as well as the practice of caregiving in both the black health-worker segment and typical black communities have been much broader than defined in conventional medical nomenclature and therapeutic practice. Local and federal public health programs and medical care institutions seeking to curtail the spread of AIDS in black populations have not on the whole planned or operated their AIDS detection and prevention programs in ways that incorporate the cultural sensitivities of black-conscious medical professionals, or the popular folk health and cultural institutions of black working-class communities.

Religious institutions, and elastic family and interpersonal arrangements remain the most effective support system in low-income black communities, with far greater behavioral influence than expensive medical care or complicated health literature. Numerous studies reveal, for example, many poor blacks still prefer spiritual churches and folk healers to (or in combination with) hospital care. Other research dealing with black female teenagers at risk for having low-birth-weight babies or infant deaths have demonstrated that a significant proportion of these teenagers will not use prenatal care programs—even services readily available to their community—when these programs lack culturally sensitive outreach procedures.[37]

In the future, if a racialist paradigm concerning black populations and AIDS susceptibility continues to grow, it will only reinforce epidemiological denial by government health agencies and the dominant American medical sector—a neglect of the critical magnitude that preventable AIDS and its deadly correlate, drug abuse, have reached throughout the black American community. Policy-making circles will downplay the social and behavioral factors that cause the disparate patterns of AIDS, while unwittingly playing up superficial skin-color manifestations of AIDS' spread in "black" and "white" populations. In the meantime, the opportunity to integrate into AIDS prevention programs the black American community's complex indigenous cultural resources—resources that have formed over decades, even centuries, and in two continents, Africa and America—will have been lost. Likewise, if new health science, social research, and care programs to control AIDS in black communities are to develop, cultural change in the organizational and planning makeup of the national and local health care agencies must take place as well.

As for the future of black communities now facing the shadow of the AIDS challenge, a black health nationalism appears to have begun to emerge. Pockets of black medical and social welfare professionals as well as grass-roots community leaders have begun to intensify their agitation for the expansion of AIDS initiatives for the black poor. This activism is aiming (1) outward at the public health and medical care establishment to pressure it to reorient and allocate more resources for black communities; and (2) inward as a catalyst to traditional black social and cultural institutions.

At the annual NMA conference in 1989 attended by some 5,000 physicians, some sessions emphasized the need for a federal commitment to expand research into the social and economic factors associated with high rates of AIDS among blacks, as well as the particular needs of black women, mothers, and infants with AIDS. They also called for the public and private researchers "to be aware of these factors in educating blacks about AIDS and in training white doctors who are working with blacks who have the virus or who are at high risk of acquiring it." Finally, NMA conferees urged toughening of federal antidiscrimination laws protecting those with AIDS.[38]

Meanwhile, alarm and frustration throughout the black community regarding the lack of more resources and education to curtail the spread of AIDS has risen. During the summer of 1988, a federal health agency attempted to begin a pilot study on the prevalence of HIV infection using blood test from households throughout neighborhoods in the District of Columbia. Once Washington residents and city officials learned of this study, their protests were so strong the study had to be scrapped. Newspapers reported that city health officials were upset that they had not been consulted about this study. Other local leaders "expressed concern that Washington's black community was being used as a 'guinea pig' in a project that would stigmatize the city and its minority communities."[39]

The growing sense of urgency throughout the lay black community regarding the AIDS crisis was summarized best by a black journalist writing on this issue in a national black magazine. "It is important for us to take a closer look at this tragic disease," he urged. "It is a matter of life and death, and could profoundly affect the survival of the Black race."[40] This outcry indicates the fixedness that racial divisions and categories hold throughout contemporary American society. It also suggests that in the future, given the history and force of racial stratification in the United States, no Americans, regardless of color, will be able to approach the dynamics of racial discriminations and the AIDS epidemic as separable problems.

Appendix

Membership List of the Conference with Negro Leaders on Wartime Problems in Venereal Disease Control, American Social Hygiene Association, 22–23 November 1943*

Bethune, Mrs. Mary McLeod
President, Council of Negro
  Women
Washington, D.C.

Bray, Bishop James A.
President, Fraternal Council of
  Negro Churches in America
Chicago, Illinois

Brown, Dr. Roscoe
Senior Health Education Specialist
U.S. Public Health Service
Washington, D.C.

Browning, Charles F.
National Representative of *Chicago
  Defender,* Chairman, Board of
  Directors, P.E.P.
(Negro Press Trade Journal)
Chicago, Illinois

Cabot, Blake
Acting Director, Public Information
  Service
American Social Hygiene Assn.
New York, N.Y.

Caliver, Ambrose
Specialist, Office of Education
Washington, D.C.

Clapp, Raymond F.
Associate Director
Social Protection Division
Federal Security Agency
Washington, D.C.

Clarke, Dr. Walter
Executive Director
American Social Hygiene Assn.
New York, N.Y.

Cornely, Dr. Paul B.
Head, Dept. of Bacteriology
Preventive Medicine and Public Health
Howard University
Washington, D.C.

Goldsmith, Judge John M.
Legal Consultant
Social Protection Division
Federal Security Agency, Chairman
Committee of Social Protection
American Bar Association
Washington, D.C.

*Source: See n.14., p. 215.

Guild, Dr. St. Clair
Director of Special Programs
National Tuberculosis Assn.
New York, N.Y.

Haynes, Dr. George
Secretary, Dept. of Race Relations
Federal Council of Churches of
     Christ in America
New York, N.Y.

Hardy, Judson
Education Officer
U.S. Public Health Service
Washington, D.C.

Heller, Dr. James R.
Asst. Surgeon General
U.S. Public Health Service
Washington, D.C.

Hinton, Dr. William A.
Boston Dispensary
Boston, Mass.

Johnson, Col. Campbell C.
Executive Assistant
Selective Service System
Washington, D.C.

Johnson, Dr. Charles S.
Director, Dept. of Social Sciences
Fisk University
Nashville, Tennessee

Johnson, Dr. Mordecai
President, Howard University
Washington, D.C.

Jones, Dr. Jesse
Director, Phelps–Stokes Fund
New York, N.Y.

Kenney, Dr. John
Superintendent, John A. Andrews
     Memorial Hospital
Editor of the *JNMA*
Tuskegee Institute, Alabama

Kinsie, Paul M.
Director of Field Studies
American Social Hygiene Assn.
New York, N.Y.

Lawless, Dr. T. K.
Dermatologist and Consultant
Provident Hospital
Chicago, Illinois

Larremore, Thomas A.
Legal Consultant
American Social Hygiene Assn.
New York, N.Y.

Lewis, Miss Vinita
Consultant in Social Services
U.S. Children's Bureau
Washington, D.C.

Love, Dr. Edgar
Director, Division of Negro
     Workers
Board of Church Missions of the
     Methodist Churches
New York, N.Y.

Mather, Philip R.
Chairman, War Activities
     Committee
American Social Hygiene Assn.
Boston, Massachusetts

Merrill, Mrs. Eleanor Brown
Executive Director, National
     Society for the Prevention of
     Blindness
New York, N.Y.

Ness, Eliot
Director, Social Protection Division
Federal Security Agency
Washington, D.C.

Paige, Judge Myles A.
Court of Special Sessions
New York, N.Y.

Poston, Theodore
Consultant, Office of War
  Information
Washington, D.C.

Price, Dr. Oma
Epidemiologist, Bureau of Social
  Hygiene
Dept. of Health
New York, N.Y.

Ragland, John M.
Specialist in Social Protection
Social Protection Division
Federal Security Agency
Washington, D.C.

Riddle, Mrs. Estelle Massey
Consultant, War Nursing Council
New York, N.Y.

Schwarta, Commander W. H.
Bureau of Medicine and Surgery
U.S. Navy
Washington, D.C.

Sengstacke, John A.
President, Negro Publishers Assn.
Managing Editor of *Chicago
  Defender*
Chicago, Illinois

Smith, Dr. T. M.
President, National Medical Assn.
Chicago, Illinois

Snow, Dr. William
Chairman, Executive Committee
American Social Hygiene Assn.
New York, N.Y.

Staupers, Mrs. Mabel K.
Executive Secretary,
National Association of Colored
  Graduate Nurses
New York, N.Y.

Turner, Lt. Col. Thomas
Chief, Venereal Disease Control
  Branch
U.S. Army
Washington, D.C.

Washington, F. B.
Director, Atlanta University School
  of Social Work
Atlanta, Georgia

Wright, Bishop R. R., Jr.
Executive Director, Fraternal
  Council of Negro Churches in
  America
Wilberforce, Ohio

Abbreviations

Repositories

ACTU   Amistad Research Center, Tulane University, New Orleans, La.
APSL   American Philosophical Society Library, Philadelphia, Pa.
FCLM   Francis A. Countway Library of Medicine, Boston Medical
           Library/Harvard Medical Library, Boston, Mass.
MSRC   Moorland-Spingarn Research Center, Howard University,
           Washington, D.C.
NLM   History of Medicine Division, National Library of Medicine,
           Bethesda, Md.
NYAM   New York Academy of Medicine, New York City, N.Y.
SLYU   Sterling Memorial Library, Manuscripts and Archives, Yale
           University, New Haven, Conn.
TUML   Tulane University Medical School Library, New Orleans, La.
UAB   Lister Hill Library of Health Sciences, University of Alabama at
           Birmingham, Birmingham, Ala.
VSL   Virginia State Library, Richmond, Va.

Medical and Public Health Periodicals

AJPH   *American Journal of Public Health*
ART   *American Review of Tuberculosis*
JAMA   *Journal of the American Medical Association*
JNE   *Journal of Negro Education*
JNMA   *Journal of the National Medical Association*
MMWR   *Morbidity and Mortality Weekly Report,* Centers for Disease
           Control, United States Public Health Service
NEJM   *New England Journal of Medicine*
PHR   *Public Health Reports,* United States Public Health Service

Notes

Introduction

1. D. R. Hopkins, "AIDS in Minority Populations in the United States," *PHR*, 102 (November–December, 1987): 677; S. R. Freidman et al., "The AIDS Epidemic Among Blacks and Hispanics," *Milbank Quarterly*, 65, supp. 2 (1987): 460–65.

2. Laura B. Randolph, "*Ebony* Interview with U.S. Surgeon General C. Everett Koop, M.D.," *Ebony*, 43 (September 1988): 155, 158.

3. Mary Gover, "Negro Mortality—III. Course of Mortality from Specific Causes, 1920–1944," *PHR*, 63, no. 7 (13 February 1948): 207–09.

4. Ibid., 208; Mary Gover, "Negro Mortality—I. Mortality From All Causes in the Death Registration States," *PHR*, 61, (22 February 1946): 259

5. See, for example, Richard F. Gillum and Kuo Chang Liu, "Coronary Heart Disease Mortality in the United States blacks, 1940–1978: Trends and Unanswered Questions," *American Heart Journal*, 108, no. 3, pt. 2 (September 1984): 729, 731.

6. See Frank F. Furstenberg, Jr., "Race Differences in Teenage Sexuality, Pregnancy, and Adolescent Childbearing," *Milbank Quarterly*, 65, supp. 2 (1987): 381–403; Alvin E. Headen, Jr., and Sandra W. Headen, "General Health Conditions and Medical Insurance Issues Concerning Black Women," *Review of Black Political Economy* 14, nos. 2–3 (Fall–Winter 1985–86): 185; Antonio A. Rene, "Racial Differences in Mortality: Blacks and Whites," in *Health Care Issues in Black America: Policy, Problems and Prospects*, edited by M. F. Rice and Woodrow Jones, Jr. (Westport, Conn.: Greenwood, 1987), 31–40; D. R. Hopkins, "AIDS in Minority Populations."

7. James Summerville, *Educating Black Doctors: A History of Meharry Medical College* (University, Ala.: University of Alabama Press, 1983); E. H. Beardsley, *A History of Neglect: Health Care for Blacks and Mill Workers in the Twentieth-Century South* (Knoxville: University of Tennessee Press, 1987).

8. Ronald L. Numbers, "The History of American Medicine: A Field in Ferment," in *The Promise of American History: Progress and Prospects*, edited by S. I. Kutler and S. N. Katz (Baltimore: Johns Hopkins University Press, 1982), 255. Since this historiographical survey, three newer works have

appeared that discuss the continuing research in black health history: E. H. Beardsley, *A History of Neglect*, 369; David McBride, *Integrating the City of Medicine: Blacks in Philadelphia Health Care, 1910–1965* (Philadelphia: Temple University Press, 1989), xvi; and K. F. Kiple, "A Survey of Recent Literature on the Biological Past of the Black," in *The African Exchange: Toward a Biological History of Black People*, edited by K. F. Kiple (Durham: Duke University Press, 1987), 7–34.

9. See, for instance, Thomas McKeown, *The Role of Medicine—Dream, Mirage or Nemesis?* (Princeton: Princeton University Press, 1979); Hubert Charbonneau and Andre Larose, eds., *The Great Mortalities: Methodological Studies of Demographic Crises in the Past* (Liege, Belgium: International Union for the Scientific Study of Population, 1979); Robert Woods and John Woodward, eds., *Urban Disease and Mortality in Nineteenth Century England* (New York: St. Martin's Press, 1984); Richard F. Evans, "Epidemics and Revolutions: Cholera in Nineteenth-Century Europe," *Past & Present*, no. 120 (August 1988): 123–46. For an excellent survey of recent biological and demographic health studies of Africans in New World slave societies, see Kiple, "A Survey of Recent Literature on the Biological Past of the Black."

10. Among the recent works that exemplify the race-centric interpretations of modern black America are Joel Williamson, *A Rage For Order: Black–White Relations in the American South Since Emancipation* (New York: Oxford University Press, 1986); and *"We the People" and Others: Duality and America's Treatment of its Racial Minorities* (London: Tavistock Publications, 1983). As for the interpretation subordinating the racial determinant to class, see two works by William J. Wilson, *The Declining Significance of Race* (Chicago: University of Chicago Press, 1978); and *The Truly Disadvantaged: The Inner City, the Underclass, and Public Policy* (Chicago: University of Chicago Press, 1987). A newer work that attempts provocatively to synthesize both interpretations is Harold Cruse's *Plural But Equal: A Critical Study of Blacks and Minorities and America's Plural Society* (New York: William Morrow, 1987).

11. Saxon Graham, the noted epidemiologist, has used the term "paradigm of disease development" to denote physical environments and social factors that evolve into individual pathology. Stephen J. Kunitz, in a valuable study of hookworm and pellegra, employed the term paradigm in a similar vein to delineate a "reductionist, biomedical" model versus a "holistic, ecological" model to comprehend these diseases. My use of the word paradigm, by contrast, is broader and pertains to the knowledge, ideas, and policy discourse that emerge in response to social, environmental, and pathological factors as well. See S. Graham, "The Sociological Approach to Epidemiology," *AJPH*, 64, no. 11 (November 1974): 1046–49; and S. J. Kunitz, "Hookworm and Pellegra: Exemplary Diseases in the New South," *Journal of Health and Social Behavior*, 29 (June 1988): 139–48.

12. Kenneth F. Maxcy and John P. Fox provide conventional definitions: "[A]n epidemic is defined by the fact that the number of cases, small or large, represents a significant excess over that expected on the basis of cumulated previous experience." (J. P. Fox, *Epidemiology: Man and Disease* [New York: Macmillan, 1970], 240); and "[a]n epidemic is commonly defined as a sudden increase in the prevalence of a disease which is more or less constantly present or endemic in a community." (K. F. Maxcy, "Principles of Epidemiology," in *Bacterial and Mycotic Infections of Man*, edited by Rene J. Dubos [Philadelphia: J. B. Lippincott, 1948], 683.)

13. Reuel A. Stallones, "To Advance Epidemiology," *Annual Review of Public Health*, 1 (1980): 71.

14. On the idea that medical systems of different societies have distinct explanatory models at the base of their healing institutions, see Arthur Kleinman, "Concepts and a Model for the Comparison of Medical Systems as Cultural Systems," *Social Science and Medicine*, 12, no.2B (1978): 85–93; Irwin Press, "Problems in the Definition and Classification of Medical Systems," *Social Science and Medicine*, 14B, no. 1 (1980): 45–57.

Chapter 1

1. John Hope Franklin, *From Slavery to Freedom: A History of Negro Americans* (New York: Alfred A. Knopf, 1980); Rayford W. Logan, *The Negro in American Life and Thought: The Nadir, 1877–1901* (New York: Dial Press, 1954); Herbert G. Gutman, *The Black Family in Slavery and Freedom, 1750–1925* (New York: Vintage, 1976); and Joel Williamson, *A Rage for Order: Black-White Relations in the American South Since Emancipation* (New York: Oxford University Press, 1986).

2. E. F. Frazier, *The Negro in the United States* (1949; New York: Macmillan, 1957), 567–69.

3. *The Health and Physique of the Negro American—Report of a Social Study made under the direction of Atlanta University; together with the Proceedings of the Eleventh Conference for the Study of the Negro Problems, held at Atlanta University, on May the 29th, 1906*, edited by W. E. B. Du Bois (Atlanta: Atlanta University Press, 1906), 65–91; Virginia Board of Health, "Morbidity and Vital Statistics [for the Year 1913]," *Virginia Health Bulletin*, 7, extra no. 1 (15 February 1915), VSL: 47–48; Frederick L. Hoffman, *The Mortality From Cancer Throughout the World* (Newark, N.J.: Prudential Press, 1915), [pamphlet], UAB, 130–31.

4. Du Bois, *The Health and Physique of the Negro*, 72. These mortality figures for 1900 covered about one-eighth of the nation's black population (ibid., 76).

5. Du Bois, *The Health and Physique of the Negro*, 73.

6. Ibid., 76.

7. Thomas McKeown, *The Role of Medicine: Dream, Mirage, or Nemesis?* (Princeton, N.J.: Princeton University Press, 1979), 32–42.

8. W. I. B. Beveridge, *Influenza: The Last Great Plague* (New York: PRODIST, 1978), 12, 20.

9. R. Koch, "The Aetiology of Tuberculosis" [1882], in *Source Book of Medical History*, compiled with notes by Logan Clendening (New York: Dover, 1942), 392–93.

10. George W. Comstock, "Tuberculosis," in *Maxcy-Rosenau—Public Health and Preventive Medicine*, edited by John M. Last (Norwalk, Conn.: Appleton-Century-Crofts, 1986), 222, 224.

11. Du Bois, *The Health and Physique of the Negro*, 66–70; quotation is from p. 69.

12. City records on deaths of blacks were recorded in major southern cities since the early nineteenth century. Baltimore, Charleston, and New Orleans began recording mortality of blacks in 1817, 1822, and 1845, respectively. (Eugene K. Jones, "The Negro's Struggle for Health," *Opportunity*, 1, no. 6 [June 1923]: 4; Mary Gover, "Trend of Mortality Among Southern Negroes Since 1920," *JNE*, 6, no.3 [July 1937]: 276).

13. Du Bois,, *The Health and Physique of the Negro*, 76.

14. Louis I. Dublin, "Vital Statistics," United States Public Health Service, *Municipal Health Department Practice for the Year 1923 Based Upon Surveys of the 100 Largest Cities in the United States, Public Health Bulletin no. 164, July 1926* (Washington, D.C.: GPO, 1926), 62–79.

15. Although during the early decades of the twentieth century physicians in private practice generally opposed most public health activities, they tended to support collection of aggregate vital statistics because this service posed no threat to their professional autonomy. George Rosen, *The Structure of American Medical Practice 1875–1941*, edited by Charles E. Rosenberg (Philadelphia: University of Pennsylvania Press, 1983), 42–43.

16. "Mortuary Report of New Orleans . . . For June, 1911," *New Orleans Medical and Surgical Journal*, 54, no. 2 (August 1911), TUML: 176. At this time, the white and black populations of New Orleans was estimated to be 272,000 and 101,000, respectively.

17. Carl V. Harris, *Political Power in Birmingham, 1871–1921* (Knoxville: University of Tennessee Press, 1977), 160–61. Although blacks composed 39 percent of Birmingham's population in 1915, they suffered 76

percent of the year's deaths from tuberculosis that occurred in this city. (Ibid.)

18. Dublin, "Vital Statistics," 63.

19. W. A. Plecker, "Report of the Registrar of Vital Statistics," *Virginia Health Bulletin*, 7, extra no. 1 (5 February 1915): VSL, 67.

20. Virginia Board of Health, "Morbidity and Vital Statistics," 48.

21. Ibid., 51. The other cities surveyed and their white and black populations were Alexandria (11,321 and 4,268), Danville (13,159 and 6,377), Lynchburg (21.232 and 10,043), Newport News (13,052 and 7,336), Petersburg (13,520 and 11,358), and Roanoke (30,302 and 8,917).

22. Ibid., 51.

23. Ibid., 49.

24. Ibid.

25. The Virginia Board of Health report, "Morbidity and Vital Statistics," contained information on infant mortality that showed rural blacks had the lowest death rates of infants below the age of two due to diarrhea and enteritis. "Country negro mothers," the report stated, "who almost always nurse their own children," had the fewest infant deaths. Black mothers of urban areas, however, who tended to nurse their infants less than rural populations and urban whites had the highest death rates in this category (58).

26. J. W. Trask, "The Significance of the Mortality Rates of the Colored Population of the United States," *AJPH*, 6, no. 3 (March 1916): 254.

27. Ibid., 254–57; quote is from p. 257.

28. Ibid., 257.

29. J. S. Fulton, "Discussion [of] 'The Significance of Mortality Rates,'" *AJPH*, 6, no. 3 (March 1916): 259–60.

30. C.-E. A. Winslow, *The Prevention of Epidemics*, [draft typescript, 14 pp.] (n.p.: c. 1950), C.-E. A. Winslow Papers–SLYU, 5; David A. Blancher, "Workshops of the Bacteriological Revolution: A History of the Laboratories of the New York City Department of Health, 1892–1912," (Ph.D. diss., City University of New York, 1979), 234–35.

31. Richard Hofstadter, *Social Darwinism in American Thought* (Philadelphia: University of Pennsylvania Press, 1944); Philip Mason, "The Revolt Against Western Values," *Color and Race*, edited by John Hope Franklin (Boston: Beacon Press, 1968), 52; Lewis Coser, "American Trends," in *A History of Sociological Analysis*, edited by Thomas Bottomore and Robert Nisbet (New York: Basic Books, 1978), 293, 298–99.

32. Alan Chase, *The Legacy of Malthus: The Social Costs of the New Scientific Racism* (Urbana: University of Illinois Press, 1980), 177–80; Daniel J. Kevles, *In The Name of Eugenics: Genetics and the Uses of Human Heredity* (New York: Alfred A. Knopf, 1985), 72.

33. Thomas F. Gossett, *Race: The History of an Idea in America* (New York: Schocken Books, 1968), 281–282; Alexander Thomas and Samuel Sillen, *Racism and Psychiatry* (Secaucus, N.J.: Citadel Press, 1979), 20–21, 34–35; Stephen J. Gould, *The Mismeasure of Man* (New York: W. W. Norton, 1981), 77–112; Williamson, *A Rage For Order,* 89.

34. F. L. Hoffman, *Race Traits and Tendencies of the American Negro,* Publication of the American Economic Association; Vol. II, nos. 1–3 (New York, 1896); and R. Matas, *The Surgical Peculiarities of the Negro, Transactions of the American Surgical Association,* 14 (1896): 483–606. Even nearly two decades after its appearance, Hoffman relied on Matas's *Surgical Peculiarities* to demonstrate blacks were relatively more immune to cancer. For an example of the impact of the works by Hoffman and Matas through the 1930s, see Isidore Cohn, "Carcinoma of the Breast in the Negro," *Annals of Surgery,* 107, no. 5 (May 1938), rpt. in *Selected Papers of Isidore Cohn, Vol. 2, 1930–1945, Medical Department, Tulane University,* [unpublished compendium], TUML, 717.

35. Gutman, *The Black Family in Slavery and Freedom,* 538. The important studies on American racial thought and research (see notes 32 and 33) detail the intellectual and political context for the "dying race" idea and influence of Hoffman and his like–minded contemporaries working in demography and sociology. However, they make no mention of Matas and his work, a subject in need of research by investigators of the historical sociology of American medical knowledge.

36. Hoffman, *Race Traits and Tendencies of the American Negro* 95, 176, 329.

37. F. L. Hoffman, "The Educational Value of Cancer Statistics to Insurance Companies, the Public and the Medical Profession," paper read before the Clinical Congress of Surgeons of North America, Chicago, 13 November 1913, *Frederick L. Hoffman, Papers On Cancer,* [unpublished compendium], Roswell Park Memorial Institute Library, Buffalo, New York, [hereafter abbreviated Hoffman Papers-RIL], 70.

38. F. L. Hoffman, "The Cancer Problem in the Southern States," address at Columbia Medical Society Cancer Meeting, 12 January 1922, Columbia, South Carolina, Hoffman Papers-RIL, 239. On the idea that the nearness to "torrid" or "semitorrid" regions was a factor in lower cancer rates, see Hoffman, "Some Essential Statistics of Cancer Mortality throughout the World," part of the Commemoration Volume issued by the American Medical Association at its meeting in San Francisco, 22–26 June 1915," Hoffman Papers-RIL, 108–09.

39. F. L. Hoffman, "The Menace of Cancer," Address delivered before the 38th annual meeting of the American Gynecological Society, Washington, D.C., 6–8 May 1913, Hoffman Papers-RIL, 23.

40. See, for instance, F. L. Hoffman, "The Menace of Cancer," *The Survey* (30 August 1913), rpt. in Hoffman Papers-RIL, 62.

41. Hoffman, "The Cancer Problem in the Southern States," 238.

42. Shufeldt, *America's Greatest Problem: The Negro* (Philadelphia: F. A. Davis, 1915).

43. Ibid., 251–52.

44. Ibid., 252.

45. C. V. Roman, *American Civilization and the Negro—The Afro-American in Relation to National Progress* (Philadephia: F. A. Davis, 1916; rpt., Northbrook, Ill.: Metro Books, 1972), 89, 120.

46. Ibid., 240.

47. In 1910 only twenty-one states and the District of Columbia recorded deaths with sufficient accuracy for inclusion in the United States Census Bureau's official death registration area. However, by 1940 this number grew so that over 94 percent of white and 82 percent of nonwhite births and deaths were within the official registration zone. United States Department of Commerce, Bureau of the Census, *Negroes in the United States* (Washington, D.C.: GPO, 1915), 43; Mary Gover, "Negro Mortality," *PHR*, 61, no. 43 (25 October 1946): 1529–30.

48. Stuart C. Gilman, "Degeneracy and Race in the Nineteenth Century: The Impact of Clinical Medicine," *Journal of Ethnic Studies*, 10, no. 4 (Winter 1983): 38–42; John H. Stanfield, *Philanthropy and Jim Crow in American Social Science* (Westport, Conn.: Greenwood Press, 1985), 25–27.

49. Quillian, "Racial Peculiarities A Cause of the Prevalence of Syphilis in Negroes," *American Journal of Dermatology & Genito-Urinary Diseases*, 10, no. 6 (June 1906): 277–79.

50. Folkes, "The Negro as a Health Problem," *JAMA*, 55, no. 15 (8 October 1910): 1246–47; T. W. Murrell, "Syphilis and the American Negro: A Medico-Sociologic Study," *JAMA*, 14, no. 11 (12 March 1910): 846–49. A similar study, Gordon Wilson's "Diseases in Apparently Healthy Colored Girls," appeared in the *New York Medical Journal*, 103, no. 13 (25 March 1916): 585–88. Wilson was a Baltimore physician.

51. Quillian, "Racial Peculiarities: A Cause of the Prevalence of Syphilis in Negroes," 277.

52. Murrell, "Syphilis and the American Negro," 846.

53. Ibid., 847.

54. Ibid.

55. Ibid.

56. G. Farrar Patton, "The Relative Immunity of the Negro to Alcoholism," *New Orleans Medical and Surgical Journal*, 64, no. 3 (September 1911), TUML: 203.

57. Henry H. Hazen, *Syphilis: A Treatise On Etiology, Pathology, Diagnosis, Prognosis, Prophylaxis, and Treatment* (St. Louis, Mo.: C. V. Mosby, 1919), 29.

58. Erwin H. Ackerknecht, *A Short History of Medicine* (Baltimore: Johns Hopkins University Press, 1982), 96–98.

59. Ibid., 180, 202; Hazen, *Syphilis*, 29; Vern L. Bullough, *Sex, Society & History* (New York: Science History Publications, 1976), 178.

60. Ackerknecht, *A Short History of Medicine*, 182; T. F. Pettigrew, *A Profile of the Negro American* (Princeton, N.J.: D. Van Nostrand, 1964), 130.

61. Ackerknecht, *A Short History of Medicine*, 181–82; Allan M. Brandt, *No Magic Bullet: A Social History of Venereal Disease in the United States Since 1880* (New York: Oxford University Press, 1987), 40.

62. During the 1910s and 1920s some medical researchers claimed that more than 50 percent of all black Americans were syphilitc. Howard Fox, "Syphilis in the Negro," *New York Medical Journal*, 26, no. 12 (15 June 1926): 555.

63. Gerald F. Pyle, *Applied Medical Geography* (Washington, D.C.: V. H. Winston & Sons, 1979), 3–4; William J. Brown et al., *Syphilis and Other Venereal Diseases* (Cambridge: Harvard University Press, 1970), 1–16.

64. Edmund C. Tramont, "Syphilis in the AIDS Era," *NEJM*, 316, no. 25 (18 June 1987): 1600.

65. Richard A. Johnson and Thomas B. Fitzpatrick, "The Skin," in *The Horizons of Health*, edited by Henry Wechsler et al. (Cambridge: Harvard University Press, 1978), 284.

66. William J. Brown, *Syphilis and Other Venereal Diseases* (Cambridge: Harvard University Press, 1970), 26–27; David Nabarro, *Congenital Syphilis* (London: Edward Arnold [1954]).

67. Norman R. Ingraham and Michael J. Burke, "Correcting the Reported Incidence of Congenital Syphilis in Philadelphia," *AJPH*, 46, no. 10 (October 1956): 1309.

68. For a review of the medical literature tracing the dispute with the concept of hereditary syphilis and the idea's subsequent decline, see Nabarro, *Congenital Syphilis*, 1–3.

69. Howard Fox, "The Anular [sic] Lesions of Early Syphilis in the Negro," *Archiv für Dermatologie und Syphilis*, 58 (1912): 315–18.

70. The serious fallacies that arise when hospital patient statistics are used to establish a general population's rate of illness are detailed in A. Bradford Crawford, *Principles of Medical Statistics* (New York: Oxford University Press, 1971), 237–43.

71. Fox, "Anular Lesions of Early Syphilis," 316.

72. Fox, "Syphilis and the Negro," 555–56.

73. Kelly Miller, *Race Adjustment—Essays on the Negro in America* (New York: Neale, 1908; rpt., New York: Arno Press and Times, 1968), 195. Dr. Williams' study "Ovarian Cysts in Colored Women" appeared in the *Philadelphia Medical Journal*, 6 (29 December 1900): 1244–48.

74. J. A. Kenney, "Health Problems of the Negroes," *Annals of the American Academy of Political and Social Science* (March 1911), rpt. in J. A. Kenney, *The Negro in Medicine* (n.p.: author, 1912), 50.

75. Ibid.

76. Roman, *American Civilization and the Negro*, 39, 40.

77. N. A., "Negro Health and Physique," in *The Health and Physique of the Negro*, edited by W. E. B. Du Bois, 13.

78. On the general scholarship of Miller and Boas regarding the race question, see R. Fred Wacker, *Ethnicity, Pluralism and Race: Race Relations Theory in America Before Myrdal* (Westport, Conn.: Greenwood, 1983), 15, 17, 22, 24–26, 29, 50–51, 79.

79. "Negro Health and Physique," 24–27; Alexander Thomas and Samuel Sillen, *Racism and Psychiatry* (Secaucus, N.J.: Citadel Press, 1979), 4–5. For a modern critique of Bean's work, see Gould, *The Mismeasure of Man*, 27, 77–82, 90, 97.

80. H. A. Miller, "Some Psychological Considerations on the Race Problem," in *The Health and Physique of the Negro*, edited by W. E. B. Du Bois, 55.

81. Miller, *Race Adjustment*, 125.

82. Miller, *The Everlasting Stain* (Washington, D.C: Associated Publishers, 1924; rpt. New York: Arno Press and Times, 1968), 200.

83. K. Miller, "The Historic Background of the Negro Physician," *Journal of Negro History*, 1, no. 2 (April 1916): 108, 109.

84. "Negro Health and Physique," 93–95.

85. Kenney, *The Negro in Medicine*.

86. Ibid., 49. Emphasis by Kenney.

87. Ibid., 48, 55.

88. Kenney, "Health Problems of the Negroes," 50.

89. Roscoe C. Brown, "The National Negro Health Week Movement," *JNE*, 6, no. 3 (July 1937): 554. Similar health campaigns were initiated by blacks in Macon and Atlanta. See John Dittmer, *Black Georgia in the Progressive Era 1900–1920* (Urbana: University of Illinois Press, 1977), 63–65.

90. Kenney, "Health Problems of the Negroes," 54–55.

91. Ibid., 55.

92. Brown, "The National Negro Health Movement," 553.

93. Ibid., 58–59; quote is by Moritz Schauz, *Der Neger in den Vereinigten Staaten von Nordamerika,* (Essen, 1911).

94. Brown, "The Nation Negro Health Week Movement."

95. Ibid.; Edward H. Beardsley, *A History of Neglect: Health Care for Blacks and Mill Workers in the Twentieth Century South* (Knoxville: University of Knoxville Press, 1987), 102–03.

96. The few hospitals that were specifically designed for patients with infectious diseases were also unpopular with physicians. As one hospital bureau official stated: "The physician's habit of speaking slurringly of the contagious disease hospitals or referring to them as pest houses does more to discourage sending patients to them than any other one thing." (Robert J. Wilson, "The Part Played by Hospitals in the Control of Contagious Diseases," *AJPH*, 6, no. 3 [March 1916]: 261).

97. Kenney, *The Negro in Medicine*, 47–48; Gladys C. Gay, "A Social Worker Looks at St. Louis," *Opportunity*, 5, no. 4 (April 1927): 113.

98. M. M. Davis, "Problems of Health Service for Negroes," *JNE*, 6, no. 3 (July 1937): 439.

99. M. F. Sloan, "The Urgent Need of Hospital Facilities for Tuberculous Negroes," *Southern Medical Journal*, 10, no. 8 (August 1917): 655.

100. Ibid., 654.

101. Ibid., 655–56.

102. Ibid., 656–57.

103. Claude A. Smith, "[Discussion of] 'The Urgent Need of Hospital Facilities,'" *Southern Medical Journal*, 10, no. 6 (August 1917): 659.

104. Paul B. Johnson (Washington, D.C.), "[Discussion of] 'The Urgent Need of Hospital Facilities,'" ibid., 660.

105. C. A. Smith, ["Discussion of] 'The Urgent Need of Hospital Facilities,'", ibid., 659.

106. R. L. Jones, "[Discussion of] 'The Urgent Need of Hospital Facilities,'" ibid., 660.

107. G. M. Tolhurst, "[Discussion of] 'The Urgent Need of Hospital Facilities,'" ibid., 659.

Chapter 2

1. Joseph R. Gusfield, *Symbolic Crusade: Status Politics and the American Temperance Movement* (Urbana: University of Illinois Press, 1963), 136; J. R. Gusfield, "Moral Passage: The Symbolic Process in Public Designations of Deviance," *Social Problems*, 15, no. 2 (Fall 1967): 175–88.

2. Helen E. Walker, *The Negro in the Medical Profession, Publications of the University of Virginia Phelps-Stokes Fellowship Papers Number Eighteen* (Charlottesville, Va.: The University, 1949), VSL, 47–49.

3. Emmett J. Scott (Special Adviser) to Dean F. Keppel (Confidential Adviser, Office of the Secretary of War), 28 February 1918, cited in Mary E. Carnegie, *The Path We Tread—Blacks in Nursing, 1854–1984* (Philadelphia: J. B. Lippincott, 1986), 165.

4. Roi Ottley and William J. Weatherby (eds.), *The Negro in New York—An Informal Social History* (New York: New York Public Library, 1967), 200.

5. Ibid.; Mabel K. Staupers, *No Time For Prejudice: A Story of the Integration of Negroes in the United States* (New York: Macmillan, 1961), 98.

6. James A. Tobey, "The Health Examination Movement," *The Nation's Health*, 5, no. 9 (September 1923): 2.

7. Surgeon General of the U.S. Army, *Annual Reports of the Surgeon General, U.S. Army to the Secretary of War* (Washington: GPO, 1918), cited in George St. J. Perrott and Dorothy Holland, "The Need for Adequate Data on Current Illness Among Negroes," *JNE*, 6, no. 3, (July 1937): 353–54; A. G. Love and C. B. Davenport, "A Comparison of White and Colored Troops in

Respect to Incidence of Disease," *Proceedings of the American Academy of Science*, 5 (1919): 66. Both penetrating and perforating wounds are serious, usually involving deep-lying body cavities or organs, and most likely are caused by knives or projectiles.

8. S. J. Holmes, *The Negro's Struggle for Survival: A Study in Human Ecology* (Berkeley: University of California Press, 1937), 81.

9. Charles H. Garvin, "Immunity to Disease Among Dark-Skinned People," *Opportunity*, 4, no. 44 (August 1926): 243.

10. S. J. Holmes, "The Principle Causes of Death Among Negroes: A General Comparative Statement," *JNE*, 6, no. 3 (July 1937): 295; H. H. Hazen, "A Leading Cause of Death: Syphilis," *JNE*, 6, no. 3 (July 1937): 310.

11. Love and Davenport, "A Comparison of White and Colored Troops in Respect to Incidence of Disease," 58–67. Davenport was a leading scientist in the American eugenics movement who studies spanned several disciplines. For a sketch of his activities and wide influence, see R. V. Guthrie, *Even the Rat Was White: A Historical View of Psychology* (New York: Harper & Row, 1976), 78–82; Daniel J. Kevles, *In The Name of Eugenics: Genetics and the Uses of Human Heredity* (New York: Alfred A. Knopf, 1985), 44–56; and Thomas F. Gossett, *Race: The History of an Idea in America* (New York: Schocken, 1968), 379, 401, 426. Love coauthored another influential study presenting racial comparisons of World War I troops along with D. C. Howard, "Influenza in the U. S. Army," *Military Surgeon*, 44 (1920), 522–58. Excerpts of Love and Davenport's study of black and white troops were distributed under the title "Where Negroes Are Immune" in the popular magazine *Literary Digest*, 72, no,. 7 (18 February 1922): 62.

12. Love and Davenport, "A Comparison of White and Colored Troops," 59, 60.

13. Gossett, *Race: The History of An Idea in America*, 373.

14. "Where Negroes Are Immune," 62.

15. E. Franklin Frazier, *The Negro in the United States* (1949; New York: Macmillan, 1957), 191.

16. Edward B. Reuter, *The American Race Problem: A Study of the Negro* (New York: Thomas Y. Crowell, 1927), 50–51. Blacks were more than one-third the population of several other southern cities: Macon, Ga. (43.6%); Augusta, Ga. (43.0%); Birmingham (39.3%); and Memphis (37.7%).

17. Editorial, "Health of Negro Mothers," *Opportunity*, 3, no. 28 (April 1925): 99.

18. Francis D. Tyson, "The Negro Migrant in the North," *Negro Migra-*

tion in 1916–1917, Reports by R. H. Leavell et al., U.S. Department of Labor, Division of Negro Economics (Washington, D.C.: GPO, 1919; rpt., New York: Negro Universities Press, 1969), 143.

19. Ibid.

20. Ibid., 144.

21. Ibid., 143; David McBride, *Integrating the City of Medicine: Blacks in Philadelphia Health Care, 1910–1965* (Philadelphia: Temple University Press, 1989), 60–62.

22. Tyson, "The Negro Migrant in the North," 143; J. H. Kerns (executive secretary, Milwaukee Urban League), "Social Service Needs in the North," *Opportunity*, 5, no. 6 (June 1927): 176. To date, these outbreaks have escaped mention, much less specific analysis, in virtually all smallpox or modern urban historiography.

23. C. St. C. Guild, "A Five-Year Study of Tuberculosis Among Negroes," *JNE*, 6, no. 3 (July 1937): 548.

24. Edwin R. Embree, "Negro Illness and Its Effect Upon the Nation's Health," *Modern Hospital*, 30, no. 4 (April 1928): 51. As for TB death rates in the major northern cities, the situation in Cleveland during 1920 is typical. That year the black mortality rate from TB reached 362 per 100,000 compared to just 83 for Cleveland's whites. K. L. Kusmer, *A Ghetto Takes Shape: Black Cleveland, 1870–1930* (Urbana: University of Illinois Press, 1976), 221.

25. I. S. Falk et al., "Tuberculosis in the City of Chicago," *Chicago's Health*, Chicago Department of Health Weekly Bulletin, edited by Herman N. Bundesen, 21, no. 26 (28 June 1927), rpt., Papers of I. S. Falk–SLYU, 170, 176–77, 179; quotation is from p. 179.

26. George W. Comstock, "Tuberculosis," in *Maxcy-Rosenau—Public Health and Preventive Medicine*, edited by John M. Last (Norwalk, Conn.: Appleton-Century-Crofts, 1986), 224. Recent medical studies have demonstrated that "the probability of infection for household contacts depended primarily on the infectiousness of the case and the intimacy of contact" (ibid.).

27. William I. Beveridge, *Influenza: The Last Great Plague* (New York: PRODIST, 1978), 31–32.

28. W. H. Frost, "Statistics of Influenza Morbidity, with Special Reference to Certain Factors in Case Incidence and Case Fatality," *PHR*, 35 (March 1920), in *Papers of Wade Hampton Frost: A Contribution to Epidemiological Method*, edited by Kenneth F. Maxcy (New York: Commonwealth Fund, 1941), 349–50; Julian H. Lewis, *The Biology of the Negro* (Chicago: University of Chicago Press, 1942), 219.

29. Lewis, *The Biology of the Negro*, 219.

30. Ibid., 217; Louis I. Dublin and Alfred J. Lotka, *Twenty-Five Years of Health Progress* (New York: Metropolitan Life Insurance Co., 1937), 134–38; Holmes, *The Negro's Struggle For Survival*, 104.

31. Frost, "Statistics of Influenza Morbidity," 350.

32. Editorial, "Mortality of Negro Mothers," *Opportunity*, 3, no. 28 (April 1925): 99.

33. F. B. Washington, "Health Work for Negro Children," *Opportunity*, 3, no. 33 (September 1925): 264–65. Washington was also a consultant to the Pennsylvania state department of welfare. The infant death rate he used was based on deaths under 1 year of age per 1,000 live births.

34. Garvin, "Immunity to Disease Among Dark-Skinned People," 245.

35. Washington, "Health Work for Negro Children," 265. Washington gives the name of the researcher, Robert Woodbury, but not the exact year or citation for this nutrition survey.

36. Ibid., 265.

37. Tyson, "The Negro Migrant in the North," 144–45.

38. Ibid., 145.

39. John Hope Franklin and Alfred A. Moss, Jr., *From Slavery to Freedom: A History of Negro Americans* (New York: Alfred A. Knopf, 1988), 313–16; quotation is from p.313.

40. C.-E. A. Winslow, "Poverty as a Factor in Disease," *National Conference of Social Work* (1919), [reprint pamphlet], C.-E. A. Winslow Papers –SLYU, 1.

41. J. J. Durrett and W. G. Stromquist, *A Study of Violent Deaths Registered in Atlanta, Birmingham, Memphis and New Orleans for the Years 1921 and 1922*, (Memphis: Department of Health, City of Memphis, [1923]), Alabama State Library, Birmingham, Alabama, 1.

42. Ibid., 6–8. As for the gender of perpetrators and victims, the report stated: "Colored women largely confine their killing to colored men and occasionally include a colored woman. White women always selected as their victims white men" (8).

43. M. W. Susser and W. Watson, *Sociology in Medicine* (New York: Oxford University Press, 1971), 12, 89–90; quotation is from p.12. See also M. L. Rosenberg et al., "Interpersonal Violence: Homicide and Spouse Abuse," in *Maxcy-Rosenau—Public Health and Preventive Medicine*, edited by J. M. Last, 1404–09.

44. K. E. Barnhart, "Negro Homicides in the United States," *Opportunity*, 10, no. 7 (July 1932): 213–14; quotation is from p. 213.

45. C. S. Johnson, "The New Frontage on American Life," in *The New Negro*, edited by Alain Locke (1925; rpt., New York: Atheneum, 1983), 285.

46. E. J. McDougald, "The Task of Negro Womanhood," in *The New Negro*, edited by Alain Locke, 382.

47. "Who's Who," *Opportunity*, 5, no. 1 (January 1927): 27. The Commission on Interracial Cooperation (which later became the Southern Regional Council headquartered in Atlanta) focused on convening black and white civic activists for educational and community reform efforts. Its chief concern was liberalizing the southern white press and eliminating lynching. Gunnar Myrdal, *An American Dilemma: The Negro Problem and Modern Democracy* (1944; New York: Harper & Row, 1962), 842–50; T. F. Pettigrew, "Introduction," *The Sociology of Race Relations: Reflection and Reform*, edited by T. F. Pettigrew (New York: Free Press, 1980), 48.

48. R. B. Eleazer, "Trends in Race Relations in 1926," *Opportunity*, 5, no. 1 (January 1927): 17.

49. H. F. Dowling, *City Hospitals—The Undercare of the Underprivileged* (Cambridge: Harvard University Press, 1982), 158–59; quotation is from p. 158.

50. V. M. Alexander and G. E. Simpson, "Negro Hospitalization," *Opportunity*, 15, no. 8 (August 1937): 231–32; quotation is from p. 232. On the local background and impact of the Alexander–Simpson study, see McBride, *Integrating the City of Medicine*, 117–22.

51. Dowling, *City Hospitals*, 158–59.

52. E. R. Embree, *Investment in People: The Story of the Julius Rosenwald Fund* (New York: Harper's, 1949), 107–08.

53. E. F. Frazier, *The Negro in the United States* (1949; New York: Macmillan, 1957), 579; Carter G. Woodson, *The Negro Professional Man and the Community With Special Emphasis on the Physician and the Lawyer* (1934; rpt. New York: Negro Universities Press, 1969), 122–23, 316–17. On the importance of folk healers as a traditional source for informal health care in the black community, see Rachel E. Spector, *Cultural Diversity in Health and Illness*, (New York: Appleton-Century-Crofts, 1979), 234; Wilbur H. Watson, "Folk Medicine and Older Blacks in Southern United States," in *Black Folk Medicine: The Therapeutic Significance of Faith and Trust*, edited by W. H. Watson (New Brunswick, N.J.: Transaction Books, 1984), 53–66; and Hans A. Baer, *The Black Spiritual Movement: A Response to Racism* (Knoxville: University of Tennessee Press, 1984). Earlier, classic works by Melville J. Herskovitz make abundant references to "the magico-medical

192

Notes

complex of the American Negro, indicating point after point at which African tradition has held fast." (M. J. Herskovitz, *The Myth of the Negro Past* [1941; rpt. Boston: Beacon, 1958], 241).

54. "Editorials—Superstition and Health," *Opportunity*, 4, no. 43 (July 1926): 206; "More About Superstitions and Health," *Opportunity*, 4, no. 45 (September 1926): 271.

55. For instance, death rates (crude) for black Americans from 1916 to 1918 rose from 19.1 to 25.6; but during 1919 to 1922 dropped from 17.9 to 15.2. (Mary Gover, "Negro Mortality," *PHR*, 61, no. 43 [22 February 1946]: 265).

56. For the importance of social factors in the multifactorial disease model of current epidemiology, see the valuable essay by G. M. Oppenheimer, "In the Eye of the Storm: The Epidemiological Construction of AIDS," in *AIDS: The Burdens of History*, edited by Elizabeth Fee and D. M. Fox (Berkeley: University of California Press, 1988), 267–300.

57. Thomas McKeown, *The Role of Medicine: Dream, Mirage or Nemesis?* (Princeton, N.J.: Princeton University Press, 1979), 12–25; R. C. Lewontin et al., *Not In Our Genes: Biology, Ideology, and Human Nature* (New York: Pantheon, 1984), 57–61.

58. E. H. Sutherland, "The Biological and Sociological Processes," in *The Urban Community: Selected Papers from the Proceedings of the American Sociological Society, 1925*, edited by E. W. Burgess (Chicago: 1926; rpt., New York: Greenwood Press, 1968), 70.

59. A. L. Harris, "Defining the Negro Problem," *Opportunity*, 3, no. 25 (January 1925): 26–27; quotation is from p. 27, emphasis by Harris.

60. Kevles, *In The Name of Eugenics*, 195–96.

61. Ella F. Grove, "On the Value of the Blood-Group Feature as a Means of Determining Racial Relationship," *Journal of Immunology*, 12, no. 4 (October 1926): 251; Reuben Ottenberg and David Beres, "The Heredity of the Blood Groups," in *The Newer Knowledge of Bacteriology and Immunology By Eighty-Two Contributors*, edited by Edwin O. Jordan and I. S. Falk (Chicago: University of Chicago, 1928), 913–14. The two key studies frequently cited as authority for the blood-group race index were: L. and H. Hirschfeld, "Serological Differences Between the Blood of Different Races," *Lancet*, 2, no. 600 (October 1919): 675–79; and R. Ottenberg, "A Classification of Human Races Based on Geographic Distribution of the Blood Groups," *JAMA*, 84, no. 19 (May 1925): 1393–95.

62. Grove, "On the Value of the Blood-Group Feature," 260.

63. See, for example, Morton C. Kahn, "A Tuberculin Survey of the

Upper Aucaner Bush Negroes in Dutch Guiana," *American Journal of Hygiene*, 24, no. 3 (November 1936): 456–77. For a summary of later blood-grouping racial classifications and critique of the misuse of blood-grouping to substantiate races, see, N. P. Dubinin, "Race and Contemporary Genetics," in *Race, Science and Society*, edited by L. C. Dunn et al. (New York: UNESCO/Columbia University Press, 1956), 68–94; and Robert Miles, *Racism and Migrant Labour* (London: Routledge & Kegan Paul, 1982), 15–21.

64. Reuter, *The American Race Problem*, 174–75.

65. Ibid., 169–70.

66. Charles S. Johnson, "A Discussion of Dr. E. B. Reuter's Paper 'Racial Research: 1930–1939, Trends, Achievements, and Methods of Research,'" [unpublished typescript, 7 pp., 1940?], Box 160, Folder 23, Charles S. Johnson Papers–ACTU, 1–2.

67. Holmes was one of the founders of the Human Betterment Foundation (1928), a group of scientists and educators that advocated pro–sterilization policies throughout California. *National Health Agencies—A Survey With Especial Reference to Voluntary Assocations* (Washington, D.C.: Public Affairs Press, 1945), 222–23. On his other professional activities in behalf of the American eugenics movement, see Kevles, *In the Name of Eugenics*, 75, 101, and 331, n.22.

68. Holmes, *The Negro's Struggle For Survival*, 212–13.

69. See, for example, Guy B. Johnson, "The Negro Migration and Its Consequences," *Social Forces*, 2 (March 1924) in *The Sociology of Race Relations*, edited by T. F. Pettigrew, 79–81.

70. L. I. Dublin, *The Reduction in Mortality Among Colored Policyholders—An Address Delivered Before the Annual Conference of the National Urban League, Newark, New Jersey, October 21, 1920* (n.p., 1920), [pamphlet], Washington Collection, Hollis Burke Frissell Library, Tuskegee Institute, Tuskegee, Alabama; quotation is from p. 2.

71. Ibid., 4–5.

72. Ibid., 6.

73. C. S. Johnson, review of *Health and Wealth*, by Louis I. Dublin (1928), in *Opportunity*, 6, no. 9 (September 1928): 276.

74. J. A. Tobey, "The Death Rates Among American Negroes," *Current History*, 25, no. 2 (November 1926): 217, 218, 219.

75. Embree, "Negro Illness and Its Effect Upon the Nation's Health," 51.

76. The period from the 1900s to the 1930s has been called the "Gold-

en Age of Nutrition" by historians of early nutrition research. (National Research Council, Commission on Life Sciences, Food and Nutrition Board, Committee on Nutrition in Medical Education, *Nutrition Education in U. S. Medical Schools* [Washington, D.C.: National Academy Press, 1985], 10).

77. E. R. Embree, "Introduction," *Human Biology and Racial Welfare*, edited by Edmund V. Cowdry (1930; rpt. College Park, Md.: McGrath, 1970), xiv.

78. J. R. Paul, *An Account of the American Epidemiological Society* (Philadelphia: Philadelphia College of Physicians and Surgeons, [c. 1974]), 55; E. D. Pellegrino, "The Sociocultural Impact of Twentieth-Century Therapeutics," in *The Therapeutic Revolution: Essays in the Social History of American Medicine*, edited by M. J. Vogel and C. E. Rosenberg (Philadelphia: University of Pennsylvania Press, 1979) 245–66.

79. Paul, *An Account of the American Epidemiological Society*, 48–50.

80. Irwin M. Braverman, *Skin Signs to Systemic Disease* (Philadelphia: W. B. Saunders, 1970), v; Paul B. Beeson et al., *Cecil Textbook of Medicine*, 15th ed. (Philadelphia: W. B. Saunders Co., 1979), 166–67, 213, 2267–312.

81. Rene and Jean Dubos, *The White Plague—Tuberculosis, Man and Society* (Boston: Little, Brown, 1952), 116–17; Walter Pagel et al., *Pulmonary Tuberculosis: Bacteriology, Pathology, Diagnosis, Management, Epidemiology, and Prevention* (London: Oxford University Press, 1964), 195–98.

82. E. L. Opie, "Active and Latent Tuberculosis in the Negro Race," *ART*, 10, no. 3 (November 1924): 265. See also by Opie, "The Epidemiology of Tuberculosis of Negroes," *ART*, 22, no. 6 (December 1930): 603–12; "Tuberculosis in Jamaica," *American Journal of Hygiene*, 12, no. 1 (July 1930): 1–61; and (with F. M. McPhedran and Persis Putnam), "The Fate of Negro Persons in Contact with Tuberculosis," *American Journal of Hygiene*, 23, no. 3 (May 1936): 515–29. For Opie's additional research papers, see "Published Papers—Eugene L. Opie," [typescript, 18 pp., n.d.], Eugene L. Opie Papers–APSL.

83. On Opie's research contributions, see Esmond R. Long, "A Pathologist's Recollections of the Treatment, Investigation, and Control of Tuberculosis," *Perspectives in Biology and Medicine*, 5, no. 1 (Autumn 1961): 38.

84. Paul, *An Account of the American Epidemiological Society*, 54.

85. [E. L. Opie?], "A Projected Investigation of the Role of Constitutional Factors in Tuberculosis, Including A Study of Tuberculosis in the Negro Race," [typescript, 7 pp., c. 1925], E. L. Opie Papers–APSL, 2. Opie's name is not affixed to this item. However, its style and location in his private papers strongly suggest Opie was its author. Also, the fact is that Opie vigorously pursued the type of race-TB research this statement called for. See n. 82 above.

86. C. J. Hatfield to M. M. Davis, 3 June 1929; M. M. Davis to C. J. Hatfield, 8 June 1929; Papers of Julius Rosenwald, Box 30, Folder 17, Special Collections, The John Regenstein Library, University of Chicago, Chicago, Illinois. Opie's research in Jamaica had been sponsored by the International Health Board of the Rockefeller Foundation.

87. E. L. Opie to Charles J. Hatfield, 12 March 1932, enclosure: "Investigation in Progress at the Henry Phipps Institute, March 11, 1932," [typescript, 4 pp.]; and "The Advisory Council of the Henry Phipps Institute—Memoramdum of Discussion at the Meeting On Saturday, May 2nd, 1936," [mimeographed, 4 pp.], quotation is from p. 3; both items in Folder: "Phipps, Henry, Institute," E. L. Opie Papers–APSL.

88. W. G. Smillie and D. L. Augustine, "Vital Capacity of the Negro Race," *JAMA*, 87, no. 25 (18 December 1926): 2055–58. For an example of the impact of this study, see S. J. Holmes, "The Principal Causes of Death Among Negroes: A General Comparative Statement," *JNE*, 6, no. 3 (July 1937): 291–92; and Louis I. Dublin, "The Problem of Negro Health as Revealed by Vital Statistics," *JNE*, 6, no. 3 (July 1937): 273–74.

89. Smillie and Augustine, "Vital Capacity of the Negro," 2055. The researchers stated: "The men of this camp were selected by the state from their state prison population, on the basis of their excellent physical condition, since the state contracted their services to the logging camp. The men were well housed, well fed and had excellent medical care. They were required to work hard, and most of them were in splendid physical condtion. Negroes and whites worked side by side, their food was the same, and all conditions of living may be considered as comparable. The methods of measurement used were the same in the groups of children and of adult men, so that one description is sufficient." (Ibid.).

90. Ibid.

91. Ibid., 2055, 2057–58; quotations are from 2057, 2058.

92. Henry H. Hazen, "Syphilis in the American Negro," *JAMA*, 63, no. 6 (8 August 1914): 464–65; H. H. Hazen, *Syphilis: A Treatise on Etiology, Pathology, Diagnosis, Prognosis, Prophylaxis, and Treatment* (St. Louis, Mo.: C. V. Mosby, 1919), 24–25.

93. Hazen, "Syphilis in the American Negro," 465.

94. Hazen, *Syphilis*, 24–25.

95. A. M. Brandt, "Racism and Research: The Case of the Tuskegee Syphilis Study," *Hastings Center Report*, 8, no. 6 (December 1978): 21–29; James H. Jones, *Bad Blood: The Tuskegee Syphilis Experiment* (New York: Free Press, 1981), 16–29.

96. Hazen, "Syphilis in the American Negro," 463.

97. H. H. Hazen, "A Leading Cause of Death Among Negroes: Syphilis," *JNE*, 6, no. 3 (July 1937) 310–12, 321; quotation is from p. 310. (Note also that in this piece Hazen capitalizes "Negro.") H. H. Hazen, *Syphilis in the Negro: A Handbook for the General Practitioner, Supplement No. 15 to Venereal Disease Information* (Washington, D.C.: GPO for United States Public Health Service/Federal Security Agency, 1942), vii–ix. For more on Hazen's application of social class and the prevalence of syphilis among blacks, see Charles S. Johnson, "Health—Mortality Trends and the Transition From Folk Medium to Scientific Medium," [unpublished typescript, 45 pp.], [1948?], Box 163, Folder 11, C. S. Johnson Papers–ACTU, 20–21.

98. McBride, *Integrating the City of Medicine*, 42–43, 45–46, 52–54, 67, 70.

99. Long, "A Pathologist's Recollections of the Treatment, Investigation, and Control of Tuberculosis," 38–39.

100. On Landis's career and local influence, see McBride, *Integrating the City of Medicine*.

101. H. R. M. Landis, "The Tuberculosis Problem and the Negro," *Virginia Medical Monthly* (January 1923), rpt. in *Sixteenth Report of the Henry Phipps Institute, 1923* (Philadelphia), 1–6.

102. Ibid., 3, 4.

103. Ibid., 4–5.

104. For an early reference to the difficulty of establishing ratios of clinical to subclinical attacks of TB, see K. F. Maxcy, "Principles of Epidemiology," in *Bacterial and Mycotic Infections of Man*, edited by Rene J. Dubos (Philadelphia: J. B. Lippincott, 1948), 685–86. The most recent view is synopsized by George W. Comstock, "Tuberculosis," in *Maxcy-Rosenau—Public Health and Preventive Medicine*, edited by J. M. Last, 224–25.

105. For an excellent technical critique of alleged genetic races by current experts, see R. C. Lewinton et al., *Not In Our Genes*.

106. McBride, *Integrating the City of Medicine*, 52–55, 66–70; Washington, "Health Work for Negro Children," 268.

107. Ira V. Hiscock et al., "Infant Hygiene," United States Public Health Service, *Municipal Health Department Practice for the Year 1923 Based Upon Surveys of the 100 Largest Cities in the United States, Public Health Bulletin no. 164, July, 1926* (Washington, D.C.: GPO, 1926), 245–46; S. C. Prescott and M. P. Horwood, *Sedgwick's Principles of Sanitary Science and Public Health* (New York: Macmillan, 1935), 510–12; Richard H. Shryock, *The Development of Modern Medicine* (Madison: University of Wisconsin Press, 1979), 329; Rosemary Stevens, *American Medicine and the Public Interest* (New Haven, Conn.: Yale University Press, 1973), 200.

108. Mayhew Derryberry, "The Significance of Infant Mortality Rates," *PHR*, 51, no. 18 (May, 1936): 545–46.

109. Harry F. Dowling, *Fighting Infection: Conquests of the Twentieth Century* (Cambridge: Harvard University Press, 1978), 64; Stevens, *American Medicine and the Public Interest*, 200; Paul Starr, *The Social Transformation of American Medicine* (New York: Basic Books, 1982), 260–61.

110. J. H. M. Knox, Jr., and Paul Zentai, "The Health Problem of the Negro Child," *AJPH*, 16, no. 8 (August 1926): 805.

111. J. H. M. Knox, Jr., "The Preschool Child in Rural Maryland," *Transactions of the Medical and Chirurgical Faculty of Maryland* (1924), cited in Knox and Zentai, "The Health Problem of the Negro Child," 809, n.13.

112. On the popular notion associating race and rickets, see Alfred F. Hess and Lester J. Unger, "The Diet of the Negro Mother in New York City," *JAMA*, 70, no. 13 (30 March 1918): 900–02.

113. Knox and Zentai, "The Health Problem of the Negro Child," 809. Among the influential new researchers on black child health was Dr. Whitbridge Williams of Johns Hopkins. During the 1920s he demonstrated that infant mortality caused by syphilis depended on the physical condition of the mother; and that black mothers were willing attendees at infant care clinics where available. (Louis I. Dublin, "The Health of the Negro—The Outlook for the Future," *Opportunity*, 6, No. 6 [July 1928], 199).

114. Miriam E. Brailey, *Tuberculosis in White and Negro Children —Volume II—The Epidemiologic Aspects of the Harriet Lane Study* (Cambridge: The Commonwealth Fund/Harvard University Press, 1958), 3, 20.

115. Sam Shapiro et al., *Infant, Perinatal, Maternal, and Childhood Mortality in the United States* (Cambridge: Harvard University Press, 1968), 190; G. W. Comstock, "Tuberculosis," *Maxcy-Rosenau—Public Health and Preventive Medicine*, edited by J. M. Last, 233.

116. George D. Cannon, "Racial Contributions to American Culture— Subject: The Contributions of the Negro in Medicine," [typewritten, 28 pp.], public lecture delivered at New York University, 20 December 1945, Louis T. Wright Papers—MSRC, 4–10; Louis T. Wright to W. A. Hinton, 20 May 1938, Louis T. Wright Papers–FCLM; G. A. Spencer, *Medical Symphony: A Study of the Contributions of the Negro to Medical Progress in New York* (New York: author, 1947), 44, 47, 48.

117. F. L. Hoffman, "The Negro Health Problem," *Opportunity*, 4, no. 40 (April 1926): 119.

118. H. L. Harris, "Some Reactions to Dr. Hoffman's Discussion," *Opportunity*, 4, no. 45 (September 1926): 291.

119. Ibid.

120. Unfortunately, a biography of Louis Wright has yet to be written. However, for a glimpse of the professional awe Wright inspired in his colleagues as well as how he single-handedly shaped many positive developments at Harlem Hospital, see references to him in his longtime associate Aubre de. L. Maynard's autobiogarphy, *Surgeons to the Poor: The Harlem Hospital Story* (New York: Appleton-Century-Crofts, 1978). For a list of Wright's technical articles, see, *Bibliography of Scientific Papers of Louis Tompkins Wright*, [typewritten, 9 pp.], L. T. Wright Papers–FCLM.

121. Although in 1928 Wright called one of Hoffman's cancer studies "admirable," by the early 1930s he signaled Hoffman out as totally misguided in his reading of black mortality patterns. Louis T. Wright, "Cancer as it Affects the Negro," *Opportunity*, 6, no. 6 (June 1928): 169; "Dr. Wright Flays Vital Statistics," *New York Amsterdam News* [1931?], and "He Raps the Experts," *The Afro-American* [Baltimore], February 13, 1932; both excerpts in E. M. Bluestone to Robert M. Cunningham, Jr., "Fifth Installment from Personal File of Dr. Louis T. Wright," May 18, 1954, entry nos. 95 and 96; and *Pittsburgh Courier*, February 13, 1932, [newspaper clipping]; both in L. T. Wright Papers–FCLM.

Chapter 3

1. Belle Davis, "The Circle For Negro Relief," *Opportunity*, 3, no. 27 (March 1925): 86–87; J. A. Tobey, "The Death Rates Among American Negroes," *Current History*, 25, no. 2 (November 1926): 219.

2. M. O. Bousfield, "Major Health Problems of the Negro," *Hospital Social Service*, 28, no. 2 (1933): 549.

3. In a public speech on the matter of black hospitals, Edwin Embree stated "for twelve million Negroes in America there are, under the most liberal rating, only ten hospitals of standards approved by the national professional associations for the practice and useful experience of Negro physicians. This is a shocking situation." Embree, "Negro Hospitals and Health—Excerpts from an Address at Dedication of New Building of Mercy Hospital, Philadelphia," (Philadelphia, [1931?]), Box III, Folder 10, 1, Papers of Julius Rosenwald, Department of Special Collections, The Joseph Regenstein Library, The University of Chicago, Chicago, Illinois [hereafter abbreviated Papers of Julius Rosenwald–UC]. On black patients in white-controlled medical facilities, see E. R. Embree, "Negro Illness and Its Effects Upon the Nation's Health," *Modern Hospital*, 30, no. 4 (April 1928): 54.

4. Commission on the Eradication of Syphilis of the National Medical Association, "Implications From the Viewpoint of the Negro Physician," in

H. H. Hazen, *Syphilis in the Negro: A Handbook for the General Practitioner, Supplement No. 15 to Venereal Disease Information* (Washington, D.C.: GPO for United States Public Health Service/Federal Security Agency, 1942), Addendum, 81.

5. Bleecker Marquette, "Helping the Negro Solve His Problem," *The Nation's Health*, 9, no. 1 (January 1927): 19–21.

6. H. R. M. Landis, "The Negro Nurse in Public Health Work," *Child Health Bulletin*, 3, no. 1 (January 1927): 18; "The Henry Phipps Institute," *Twentieth Report of the Henry Phipps Institute—1928*, 9.

7. Landis, "The Negro Nurse in Public Health Work," 20.

8. Ira V. Hiscock, *Merriam Memorial Survey of Tuberculosis Control in Cleveland, Ohio for the Year 1930: A Survey of the Program for the Prevention and Treatment of Tuberculosis in Cleveland* (Cleveland: Anti-Tuberculosis League/Director of Public Health and Welfare, c. 1931), TUML.

9. Ibid., 34–35, 50, quotation is from p. 35; W. B. Gwinnell, "Shifting Populations in Great Northern Cities," *Opportunity*, 6, no. 9 (September 1928): 279.

10. Ira V. Hiscock, "The Development of Neighborhood Health Services in the United States," *Milbank Memorial Fund Quarterly*, 13, no. 1 (January 1935): 40.

11. F. B. Washington, "Health Work for Negro Children," *Opportunity*, 3, no. 33 (September 1925), 267. In 1925, 14,575 white infants and 3,381 black infants were born. Of the white babies, 992 died compared to 402 of the blacks. Although blacks were only about one-seventh of Baltimore's total population, black infant deaths were about one-third of such deaths in the city generally. ("Negro Mortality in Baltimore," *Opportunity*, 4, no. 46 [October 1926]: 303.)

12. Washington, "Health Work for Negro Children," 267–68; "Survey of the Month—Christmas Seals," *Opportunity*, 6, no. 12 (December 1928): 383.

13. Washington, "Health Work for Negro Children," 268–69. The Maternity and Infancy Act of 1921, or the so-called Sheppard-Towner Act, was legislation developed by the Children's Bureau to reduce maternal mortality throughout the nation. It granted federal funds to states to support health services for mothers and children. (See, Sam Shapiro et al., *Infant, Perinatal, Maternal, and Childhood Mortality in the United States* [Cambridge: Harvard University Press, 1968], 224; and Joyce Antler and D. M. Fox, "The Movement toward a Safe Maternity: Physician Accountability in New York City, 1915–1940," in *Sickness and Health in America: Readings in the History of Medicine and Public Health*, edited by J. W. Leavitt and R. L. Numbers [Madison: University of Wisconsin Press, 1978], 376–77).

14. Washington, "Health Work for Negro Children," 268.

15. On the Julius Rosenwald Fund generally, see Edwin R. Embree, *Investment in People: The Story of the Julius Rosenwald Fund* (New York: Harper's, 1949); Horace Mann Bond, *Negro Education in Alabama: A Study in Cotton and Steel* (1939; rpt. New York: Atheneum, 1969), 274–86.

16. Embree, *Investment in People*, 108.

17. Minutes of the Julius Rosenwald Fund, 16 November 1929, Addendum, Box 2, Folder 6, Papers of Julius Rosenwald–UC, 22–23; Thomas Parran, *Shadow on the Land* (New York: Reynal and Hitchcook, 1937), 161; Monroe N. Work, ed., *Negro Year Book: An Encyclopedia of the Negro, 1937–1938* (Tuskegee Institute, Ala.: Tuskegee Institute, 1938), 189–90.

18. Minutes of the Julius Rosenwald Fund, 11 May 1929, Papers of the Julius Rosenwald Fund–UC, Box 2, Folder 5, 37.

19. W. L. Warner, "American Caste and Class," *American Journal of Sociology*, 42, no. 2 (September 1936): 234–37; E. F. Frazier, *Race and Culture Contacts in the Modern World* (Boston: Beacon, 1957), 269–87.

20. L. I. Dublin and A. J. Lotka, *Twenty-Five Years of Health Progress* (New York: Metropolitan Life Insurance Company, 1937), 371; William J. Brown et al., *Syphilis and Other Venereal Diseases* (Cambridge: Harvard University Press, 1970), 61–65.

21. Minutes of the Julius Rosenwald Fund, 11 May 1929, 37–44; Minutes of the Julius Rosenwald Fund, 16 November 1929, Addendum, 22–23.

22. L. J. Usilton, "Trend of Syphilis and Gonorrhea in the United States Based on Treated Cases," *Venereal Disease Information*, 16, no. 5 (May 1935): 147–65; James H. Jones, *Bad Blood: The Tuskegee Syphilis Experiment* (New York: Free Press, 1981), 50–52; Bousfield, "Major Health Problems of the Negro," 546. This survey was part of the Health Section of the League of Nation's international investigation on the treatment and impact of syphilis.

23. R. A. Vonderlehr, "Cooperative Clinical Studies of the Treatment of Syphilis in the United States," *Milbank Memorial Fund Quarterly*, 13, no. 1 (January 1935): 133–45; Allan M. Brandt, *No Magic Bullet: A Social History of Venereal Disease in the United States Since 1880* (New York: Oxford University Press, 1987), 130–31. Treatment for (and retesting of) a syphilitic patient tended to be a long, expensive procedure that usually lasted more than a year.

24. Minutes of the Julius Rosenwald Fund, 11 May 1929, 38; Edward H. Beardsley, *A History of Neglect: Health Care for Blacks and Mill Workers in the Twentieth Century South* (Knoxville: University of Tennessee Press, 1987), 116–17.

25. Minutes of the Julius Rosenwald Fund, 11 May 1929, 42–43; Minutes of the Julius Rosenwald Fund, 16 November 1929, Addendum, 22–23. The Tennessee TB study was done with personnel and additional funds supplied by the Public Health Service and the NTA, and conducted locally by the Tennessee State Department of Health and Fisk University. One publication from this project is Elbridge Sibley, *Differential Mortality in Tennessee, 1917–1928 / A Statistical Study Conducted Jointly by the Tennessee State Department of Public Health and Fisk University* (Nashville: Fisk University Press, 1930).

26. Embree, "Negro Illness and Its Effects Upon the Nation's Health," 49–54; M. N. Work, ed., *Negro Year Book: 1937–1938*, 189–90.

27. M. O. Bousfield, "An Account of Physicians of Color in the United States," *Bulletin of the History of Medicine*, 17, no. 1 (January 1945): 82; Beardsley, *History of Neglect*, 116.

28. Minutes of the Julius Rosenwald Fund, 11 May 1929, 43–44; M. O. Bousfield, "The Adventure of Public Health Nursing," [1932?] rpt., Box 10, Folder 42, Louis T. Wright Papers–MSRC.

29. "Census of Public Health Nursing in United States," *Public Health Nurse*, 18, no. 5 (May 1926): 266; Dorothy Deming, "The Negro Nurse in Public Health," *Opportunity*, 15, no. 11 (November 1937): 333.

30. D. Deming, "The Negro Nurse in Public Health," 333.

31. H. R. M. Landis, "The Clinic for Negroes at the Henry Phipps Institute," *Transactions of the National Tuberculosis Association*, 17 (1921): 430.

32. Bousfield, "Adventure of Public Health Nursing," 6.

33. Landis, "The Negro Nurse in Public Health Work," 19–20.

34. Bousfield, "Adventure of Public Health Nursing," 6.

35. L. I. Dublin, "The Health of the Negro—The Outlook for the Future," *Opportunity*, 6, no. 7 (September 1928): 199.

Chapter 4

1. Roscoe C. Brown, "Negro Health IS a Problem," *Opportunity*, 19, no. 6 (June 1941): 165.

2. Committee on Tuberculosis Among Negroes, *A Five-Year Study and What It Has Accomplished* (New York: National Tuberculosis Association, 1937), cited in Julian H. Lewis, *The Biology of the Negro* (Chicago: University of Chicago Press, 1942), 137–138; C. St. C. Guild, "A Five-Year Study of

Tuberculosis Among Negroes," *JNE*, 6, no. 3 (July 1937): 548; George G. Ornstein, "The Leading Causes of Death Among Negroes: Tuberculosis," *JNE*, 6, no. 3 (July 1937): 303–04.

3. C. H. Garvin, "White Plague and Black Folk," *Opportunity*, 8, no. 8 (August 1930): 233.

4. F. P. Allen, "Physical Impairment Among One Thousand Negro Workers," *American Journal of Public Health and The Nation's Health*, 14, no. 6 (June 1932): 585.

5. Ira De A. Reid and J. A. Kenney, dir. "Keeping Healthy," in *The Negro in New Jersey—A Report of a Survey by the Interracial Committee of the New Jersey Conference of Social Work in Cooperation with the State Department of Institutions and Agencies* (n..p.: New Jersey Conference of Social Work, 1932), New Jersey State Library, Trenton, New Jersey, 41.

6. Winfred B. Nathan, "Health Education in Negro Public Schools," *JNE*, 6, no. 3 (July 1937): 524; Charles H. Garvin, "White Plague and Black Folk," *Opportunity*, 8, no. 8 (August 1930): 233.

7. Beatrice A. Myers and Ira De A. Reid, "The Toll of Tuberculosis Among Negroes in New Jersey," *Opportunity*, 10, no. 9 (September 1932): 279.

8. Ira V. Hiscock, *Merriam Memorial Survey of Tuberculosis Control in Cleveland, Ohio for the Year 1930: A Survey of the Program for the Prevention and Treatment of Tuberculosis in Cleveland* (Cleveland: Anti-Tuberculosis League/Director of Public Health and Welfare, c. 1931), TUML, 36. These are 1929 mortality figures.

9. F. Maurice McPhedran to Ludwig Kast, 10 April 1934, Eugene L. Opie Papers–APSL. McPhedran was a researcher at the Phipps Institute and Kast, president of the Josiah Macy, Jr. Foundation.

10. Mary Gover, "Trend of Mortality Among Southern Negroes Since 1920," *JNE*, 6, no. 3 (July 1937): 282–88.

11. Athilia E. Siegmann, "A Classification of Sociomedical Health Indicators: Perspectives for Health Administrators and Health Planners," in *Socio-Medical Health Indicators*, edited by Jack Elinson and A. E. Siegmann (Farmingdale, N.Y.: Baywood, 1977), 199.

12. Gover, "Trend of Mortality Among Southern Negroes," 285–86; Paul B. Beeson et al., *Cecil Textbook of Medicine*, 15th ed. (Philadephia: W. B. Saunders, 1979), 1387.

13. H. H. Hazen, "A Leading Cause of Death Among Negroes: Syphilis," *JNE*, 6, no. 3 (July 1937): 310–12; George St. J. Perrott and Dorothy F. Holland, "The Need for Adequate Data on Current Illness Among Negroes," *JNE*, 6, no. 3 (July 1937): 350–63; "In This Issue," *Milbank Memo-*

rial Fund Quarterly, 16, no. 1 (January 1938): 3; D. F. Holland and G. St. J. Perrott, "Health of the Negro," *Milbank Memorial Fund Quarterly*, 16, no. 1 (January 1938): 5–38.

14. Elizabeth C. Tandy, "Infant and Maternal Mortality Among Negroes," *JNE*, 6, no. 3 (July 1937): 330, 332, 348.

15. Ibid., 331–32; Brown, "Negro Health IS a Problem," 166.

16. L. I. Dublin, "The Problem of Negro Health as Revealed by Vital Statistics," *JNE*, 6, no. 3 (July 1937): 269. Dublin admitted that the data of Metropolitan Life Insurance Company tended to reflect employed, urban black populations outside the rural South. See also Brown, "Negro Health IS a Problem," 166.

17. Gover, "Trend of Mortality Among Southern Negroes Since 1920," 288.

18. Tandy, "Infant and Maternal Mortality Among Negroes," 337.

19. For a review of current medical literature on the etiology and epidemiology of occupational diseases, see Judith Areen et al., (eds.), *Law, Science and Medicine* (Mineola, N.Y.: Foundation Press, 1984), Pts. II and III; Arthur L. Frank, ed., "Section Three—Environmental Health," *Maxcy-Rosenau—Public Health and Preventive Medicine*, edited by John M. Last et al. (Norwalk, Conn.: Appleton-Century-Crofts, 1986), 495–950.

20. George St. J. Perrott, *The National Health Survey: Scope and Method of the Nation-wide Canvass of Sickness in Relation to its Social and Economic Setting*, PHR, 54, no.37 (15 September 1939), Rpt. no. 2098, 2–3; George St. J. Perrott and D. F. Holland, "The Need for Adequate Data on Current Illness Among Negroes," *JNE*, 6, no. 3 (July 1937): 353, 361–63; Clark Tibbitts, "The Socio-Economic Background of Negro Health Status," *JNE*, 6, no. 3 (July 1937): 413–28. On the growth of government surveillance of occupational risk following World War II, see W. W. Lowrance, *Of Acceptable Risk: Science and the Determination of Safety* (Los Altos, Calif.: William Kaufman, 1976).

21. Perrott and Holland, "The Need for Adequate Data," 352–63. The population surveyed covered about 7,500 white low-income families in Baltimore, Cleveland, New York (Lower East Side), Pittsburgh, Brooklyn, Detroit, Birmingham, and Syracuse, as well as 1,300 black families residing in Harlem.

22. Holland and Perrott, "Health of the Negro," 5–7, 14; quotation is from p. 14. For a recent, more precise study on the connections between excess disability of blacks with occupational risks and injuries, see J. C. Robinson, "Trends in Racial Inequality and Exposure to Work-Related Hazards,1968–1986," *Millbank Quarterly*, 65, supp. 2 (1987): 404–20.

23. L. I. Dublin, *Twenty-Five Years of Health Progress* (New York: Metropolitan Life Insurance Company, 1937), 371.

24. Ray Lyman Wilbur and Arthur M. Hyde, *The Hoover Policies* (New York: Charles Scribner's, 1937), 62. On Hoover's broad activity to limit government, even at the expense of alienating blacks from the national Republican Party, see Gunnar Myrdal, *An American Dilemma: The Negro Problem and Modern Democracy* (1944; New York: Harper & Row, 1962), 478–79; W. E. B. Du Bois, "Postscript," *Crisis*, 36, no. 5 (May 1929): 167–68; Du Bois, "Postscript," *Crisis*, 37, no. 6 (June 1931): 207–08.

25. Wilbur's impact on national medical policy can be traced in Henry E. Sigerist, "Towards A Renaissance of the American Spa," in *Henry E. Sigerist on the Sociology of Medicine*, edited by Milton I. Roemer and James M. Mackintosh (New York: MD Publications, 1960), 253; Rosemary Stevens, *American Medicine and the Public Interest* (New Haven, Conn.: Yale University Press, 1973), 209–10, 211; Paul Starr, *The Social Transformation of American Medicine* (New York: Basic Books, 1982), 261, 264, 266, 307; Victoria A. Harden, *Inventing the NIH: Federal Biomedical Research Policy 1887–1937* (Baltimore, Md.: Johns Hopkins University Press, 1986), 125, 140–41, 148. For a brief biographical sketch, see Martin Kaufman et al., eds., *Dictionary of American Medical Biography, Volume II* (Westport, Conn.: Greenwood Press, 1984), 804–05.

26. See Wilbur's statements in *The Memoirs of Ray Lyman Wilbur 1875–1949*, edited by E. E. Robinson and P. C. Edwards (Stanford, Calif.: Stanford University Press, 1961), 476–78; and Wilbur's essay, "The Health Status and Health Education of Negroes in the United States," *JNE*, 6, no. 3 (July 1937): 572–77.

27. Ray Lyman Wilbur, "Negro Cooperation in the White House Conference," *Opportunity*, 8, no. 11 (November 1930): 328–29, 344; quotations are from p. 328. Editorial, "The White House Conference," *Opportunity*, 9, no. 1 (January 1931): 6.

28. Blacks attending sessions included Eugene Kinckle Jones and T. Arnold Hill of the National Urban League; Mrs. H. R. Butler, president of the National Congress of Colored Parents and Teachers; Janie Porter Barrett, superintendent of the Virginia Industrial School; Anna E. Murray, chairman of the National Legislation Committee, National Association of Colored Women; Fannie C. Williams of the New Orleans school system; Althea H. Washington of Howard University; and Ernest T. Atwell of the National Recreation Association. (Wilbur, "Negro Cooperation in the White House Conference," 329.)

29. *Official Proceedings of the White House Conference on Child Health and Protection, Supplement to the United States Daily, 5, no. 228, Section 11 (November 28, 1930), [General Statement]*, Box 110, Folder 212,

Papers of the Bureau of Social Hygiene, Rockefeller Archive Center, Pocantico, New York, 12.

30. Ibid.

31. James A. Hamilton, *Patterns of Hospital Ownership and Control* (Minneapolis: University of Minnesota Press, 1961), 8–9; Stevens, *American Medicine and the Public Interest*, 146, n.37.

32. *White House Conference On Child Health [General Statement]*, 12.

33. Ibid., 45.

34. Ibid.

35. Stewart succeeded Mary McLeod Bethune, one of the nation's most powerful black leaders, as president of the Association. Stewart's presidency followed ten years in different offices for this organization, including four years as chairman of the Social Science Department. Throughout the Depression, Stewart's political philosophy focused on family betterment and racial self–reliance. "Survey of the Month—Women," *Opportunity*, 6, no. 12 (December 1928): 383; Paula Giddings, *When and Where I Enter: The Impact of Black Women on Race and Sex in America* (New York: Bantam Books, 1985), 204.

36. *White House Conference on Child Health [General Statement]*, 44, 45.

37. Editorial, "The White House Conference," 6. On the general "letdown" experienced by black Americans, Indians and other economically troubled public segments toward Hoover, see Ralph J. Bunche, *The Political Status of the Negro in the Age of FDR*, [1944], edited by Dewey W. Grantham (Chicago: University of Chicago Press, 1973); Joan Hoff-Wilson, "Herbert Hoover: The Popular Image of an Unpopular President," in *Understanding Herbert Hoover: Ten Perspectives*, edited by Lee Nash (Stanford, Calif.: Hoover Institution Press/Stanford University, 1987), 1–23; and W. G. Robbins, "Indian Reformers Under Attack: The Failures of Administrative Reform," in *Understanding Herbert Hoover*, 165–89.

38. Ira V. Hiscock, "The Development of the Neighborhood Health Services in the United States," *Milbank Memorial Fund Quarterly*, 13, no. 1 (January 1935): 50–51.

39. Ibid., 49; M. M. Torchia, "The Tuberculosis Movement and the Race Question, 1890–1950," *Bulletin of the History of Medicine*, 49, no. 2 (Summer 1975): 156–58. Of the eight TB sanitoriums operating in Maryland during 1932, only one, Henryton Sanitorium, provided beds for black consumptives. (William B. Mathews, "The Beginning of the Tuberculosis Movement in Maryland," [1932], rpt. in *Maryland State Medical Journal*, 25, no. 8 [August 1976]: 28–31).

40. B. T. Baggott, "Bureau of Tuberculosis," *City of Baltimore, One Hundred and Nineteenth Annual Report of the Health Department—1933*, 86.

41. James Ford, *Slums and Housing With Special Reference to New York City—History, Conditions, Policy and An Appendix Mainly Architectural by I. N. Phelps Stokes* (1936; rpt., Westport, Conn.: Negro Universities Press, 1971), 363; New York Tuberculosis and Health Association, "What You Can Do To Control Tuberculosis," [mimeographed, 4 pp., c. 1934], E. L. Opie Papers–APSL, 1.

42. "What You Can Do To Control Tuberculosis," 2.

43. Ibid.; Henry O. Harding, "Health Opportunities in Harlem," *Opportunity*, 4, no. 48 (December 1926): 386–87, quotation is from p. 387; [Winfred B. Nathan], *Health Conditions in Northern Harlem, 1923–1927 —National Tuberculosis Assocation Social Research Series, no. 2*, (n.p.: National Tuberculosis Association, 1932), 54–55; *Twenty-Five Years and Looking Forward—Program of Events Celebrating the 25th Anniversary of the Harlem Tuberculosis and Health Committee* (n.p.: [1947]), Louis T. Wright Papers–MSRC, 7–8.

44. Ibid.; quotations are from, respectively, Harding, "Health Opportunities in Harlem," 387; and [Nathan], *Health Conditions in North Harlem*, 55.

45. In 1930, the Committee on Administrative Practice of the American Public Health Association, jointly with leading health officials from major cities nationwide, rated Cleveland's TB control program among the highest in the United States. (Hiscock, *Merriam Memorial Survey of Tuberculosis in Cleveland*, 13).

46. Ibid., 47–49, 85.

47. Ibid., 32.

48. Michael M. Davis, "Problems of Health Service for Negroes," *JNE*, 6, no. 3 (July 1937): 447.

49. C. H. Payne to C. A. Barnett, 28 September 1937, *The Claude A. Barnett Papers: The Associated Negro Press, 1918–1967, Part Three, Subject File on Black Americans, 1918–1967, Series E, Medicine, 1927–1965*, edited by August Meier and Elliot Rudwick (Frederick, Md.: University Publications of America, 1986), [Microfilm], Reel 2.

50. Eugene L. Opie et al., "The Relative Frequency of Clinically Manifest Tuberculosis, Open Tuberculosis, Asymptomatic Lesions and Deaths in White and Negro Persons," *ART*, 23, no. 3 (May 1936): 536.

51. See especially F. R. Everett, "The Pathological Anatomy of Pulmonary Tuberculosis in the American Negro and the White Race," *ART*, 27,

no. 5 (May 1933): 411–64 (Everett was a Phipps researcher); M. Pinner and J. A. Kasper, "Pathological Peculiarities of Tuberculosis in the American Negro," *ART*, 26, no. 5 (November 1932): 463–91. For a concise overview of the medical literature on racial susceptibility through the mid-1930s, see James A. Doull, "Comparative Racial Immunity to Diseases," *JNE*, 6, no. 3 (July 1937): 429–37; as well as Lewis, *The Biology of the Negro*.

52. Pinner and Kasper, "Pathological Pecularities of Tuberculosis in the American Negro," cited by George G. Ornstein, "The Leading Causes of Death Among Negroes: Tuberculosis," *JNE*, 6, no. 3 (July 1937): 305.

53. R. Pearl, "The Weight of the Negro Brain," *Science*, 80, no. 2080 (9 November 1934): 431–34, rpt. in *Collected Papers from the Department of Biology of the School of Hygiene and Public Health of The Johns Hopkins University*, 11 (1935), 1–8; quotation is from p. 1.

54. On Bean's work and influence, and the constant academic disputes it provoked, see Lewis, *The Biology of the Negro*, 78–81; and Stephen J. Gould, *The Mismeasure of Man* (New York: W. W. Norton, 1981), 77–82, 97. Vint's study of body size in Kenya appeared in the *Journal of Anatomy*, 68, second part (January 1934): 216–223. Description of some of Vint's other studies of racial anatomy are found in Lewis, *The Biology of the Negro*.

55. Pearl, "The Weight of the Negro Brain," 1.

56. Ibid., 7–8.

57. S. J. Holmes, "The Principal Causes of Death Among Negroes: A General Comparative Statement," *JNE*, 6, no. 3 (July 1937): 291–92; quotation is from p. 292. It may appear ironic that this black-controlled scholarly publication would include Holmes's study. But during this period when university faculties were strictly segregated, black academic and social welfare periodicals frequently published investigations of blacks by white experts to inform their black readership of studies that were particularly derogatory of blacks and could mislead the larger white academic and political public. Usually alongside such studies by prominent white academics, the editors published opposing ones.

58. Myrdal, *An American Dilemma*, 142.

59. Holmes, "The Principal Causes of Death," 292, 294.

60. S. J. Holmes, *The Negro's Struggle for Survival: A Study in Human Ecology* (Berkeley: University of California Press, 1937), 48. For a review by a black medical comtemporary that attempted to rebut Holmes's arguments, see W. Montague Cobb, "Negro Survival," *JNE*, 7, no. 4 (October 1938): 564–66.

61. I. I. Lemann, "A Study of Disease in the Negro," *Southern Medical*

Journal, 27, no. 1 (January 1934): 33–38. In this study, Dr. Lemann gave an overview of what he asserted were definite anatomical peculiarities of Negroes. Lemann cited Holmes as his chief authority throughout this study. In conclusion, Lemann stated: "My thesis has been that the study of disease in the negro is profitable not only for the sake of helping him and delivering him from many of his woes, but also by reason of the many clues leading to the cause and control of disease in all human kind. . . . It is alluring and will be profitable to speculate further upon how much of the negro's reaction to disease is different from the Caucasian because of native endowments, structural and functional" (38).

62. William Coleman, *Yellow Fever in the North: The Methods of Early Epidemiology* (Madison: University of Wisconsin, 1987).

63. Garvin, "White Plague and Black Folk," 233.

64. Lewis, *The Biology of the Negro*, 139.

65. Myers and Reid, "The Toll of Tuberculosis Among Negroes in New Jersey," 279.

66. *Past, Present and Future Activities of the Manhattan Medical Society—A Brief Review of Major Events and a Forecast, Pamphlet no. 3* (New York: The Society, 1935), Louis T. Wright Papers–FCLM, 8–9.

67. Lewis, *The Biology of the Negro*, 135–36.

68. Ornstein, "The Leading Causes of Death Among Negroes," 305–09; quotations are from 307–08.

69. Ibid., 308.

70. Ford, *Slums and Housing With Special Reference to New York City*, 381–97; quotations are from pp. 381, 397.

71. C. R. Rein and Marguerite LeMoine, "The Relation of Syphilis to Life Insurance," *Abstract of the Proceedings of the Forty-Fifth Annual Meeting of the Association of Life Insurance Medical Directors of America, Vol. 21* (New York: Recording & Statistical Corp., 1935), NLM, 13–15; Dublin, *Twenty-Five Years of Health Progress*, 371.

72. F. O. Reinhard, "Bureau of Venereal Diseases," *City of Baltimore, One Hundred and Nineteenth Annual Report of the Health Department—1933*, 98–99.

73. Ibid., 95–97; quotations are from p. 97. On the early-twentieth-century origins of slum conditions including poor housing and health services in these areas, see Garret Power, "Apartheid Baltimore Style: The Residential Segregation Ordinances of 1910–1913," *Maryland Law Review*, 42 (1983): 289–95.

74. Reinhard, "Bureau of Venereal Diseases," 99.

75. This is one of the central interpretations in Allan M. Brandt, *No Magic Bullet: A Social History of Venereal Disease in the United States Since 1880* (New York: Oxford University Press, 1987).

76. Reinhard, "Bureau of Venereal Diseases," 99.

77. Elizabeth Fee, "Sin versus Science: Venereal Disease in Twentieth-Century Baltimore," in *AIDS: The Burdens of History*, edited by Elizabeth Fee and D. M. Fox (Berkeley: University of California Press, 1988), 127, 128.

78. Reinhard, "Bureau of Venereal Disease," 99. During the mid-1920s black social workers were employed to investigate the health problems throughout the city's poorer black sections. As the *Opportunity* editors noted in 1926, Baltimore's city and health leadership were demonstrating "[s]omething other than polite regrets and dismal predictions of ultimate termination was needed." These city leaders were "beginning to value the coldly direct methods of skilled Negro social workers." "Negro Mortality in Baltimore," *Opportunity*, 4, no. 46 (October 1926): 303.

79. Reinhard, "Bureau of Venereal Diseases," 99–100.

80. R. A. Vonderlehr, "Cooperative Clinical Studies of the Treatment of Syphilis in the United States," *Milbank Memorial Fund Quarterly*, 13, no. 1 (January 1935): 134.

81. On how mainstream sexual values constrained federal and municipal campaigns against venereal disease in post-Depression America, see the valuable studies by Brandt, *No Magic Bullet*; and Fee, "Sin versus Science." As for the broad importance attached to the study of disease in blacks generally, see n. 61 above. Also, Thomas Parran's popular book on the anti-VD campaign, *Shadow on the Land* (New York: Reynal & Hitchcock, 1937), listed eight questions underlying the studies of Southern rural blacks: "(1) What is the incidence of syphilis as shown by the Wassermann tests among the rural negro population of all ages? (2) Can rural negroes be induced to accept Wassermann tests and those with syphilis induced to take an amount of treatment sufficient to render them noninfectious? (3) Can satisfactory treatment of syphilis be given under field conditions? (4) Can these special activities for syphilis control be integrated with the general health program of the community? (5) At what cost can the case-finding and treatment methods be carried out? (6) To what extent can funds be secured from state and local tax sources to bear the cost of this project? (7) What are the direct and indirect effects of syphilis upon these negro populations in terms of sickness and death? And finally, the most important question, (8) Can syphilis be controlled by these intensive medical methods; and if so, how soon and at what rate can its prevalence be reduced?" (161–62). Thus, intensifying the Public Health Service's research questions concerning racial

factors and syphilis (nos. 1, 2, and 7) were matters related to maintaining a healthy rural black workforce (no. 3), and the costs and resources required (nos. 5 and 6).

82. Myrdal described anti-amalgamation as the doctrine of the biological, psychological, and cultural inferiority of blacks, which was the underpinning of the powerful social and legal sanctions against integrated institutions and intermarriage. See Myrdal, *An American Dilemma*, 50–80.

83. For an account of the rise of government sponsored research as the dominant force in the nation's battle against cancer from the 1920s through the 1940s, see James T. Patterson, *The Dread Disease: Cancer and Modern American Culture* (Cambridge: Harvard University Press, 1987), 114–70.

84. Roscoe C. Brown, "The National Negro Health Week Movement," *JNE*, 6, no. 3 (July 1937): 559–60.

85. Roscoe C. Brown, "The National Negro Health Week Movement," *Health Officer*, 206 (October 1936): 7–8; Thomas Parran, "A General Introductory Statement of the Problems of the Health Status and Health Education of Negroes," *JNE*, 6, no. 3 (July 1937): 266–67.

86. K. W. Deutsch, *Nationalism and Its Alternatives* (New York: Alfred A. Knopf, 1969), 14. See also Deutsch, *Nationalism and Social Communication* (Cambridge: M. I. T. Press, 1966).

87. Parran, "General Introductory Statement," 265.

88. On the general growth of the cultural authority of medicine, see Starr, *The Social Transformation of American Medicine*; K. G. Johnson, "Reaching Out to the Community: Responses by Medicine," *Daedalus— America's Doctors, Medical Science, Medical Care*, 115, no. 2 (Spring 1986): 163–65.

89. Harden, *Inventing the NIH*, 97.

90. No recent systematic study of the early-twentieth-century African-American folk health system yet exists. For a sense of the strength and complexity of this institution in pre–World War II black America, see material in Richard M. Dorson, *American Negro Folktales* (1956; New York: Fawcett, 1967); and John Bennett, *The Doctor of the Dead: Grotesque Legends & Folk Tales of Old Charleston* (New York: Rinehart, 1946). An important new study of midwifery in the South based on interviews with traditional black midwives is Debra Anne Susie's, *In the Way of Our Grandmothers: A Cultural View of Twentieth-Century Midewifery in Florida* (Athens, Ga.: University of Georgia Press, 1988). On black folk health care and the therapeutic function of black churches, see the studies discussed in Chapter 2, n. 53.

91. Katharine F. Lenroot, "The Health Education Program of the Children's Bureau, with Particular Reference to Negroes," *JNE*, 6, no. 3 (July 1937): 509.

92. "Presidential Address by Peyton F. Anderson, M. D.," April, 1934, [typewritten, 9 pp.], Folder 15, Box 130-10, Louis T. Wright Papers–MSRC, 6–7.

93. Parran, *Shadow on the Land*, 165.

94. Parran, "General Introductory Statement," 266.

95. Ibid., 267, emphasis mine.

96. T. Parran, "The Control of Syphilis," *Venereal Disease Information*, 18, no. 7 (July 1937): 226.

97. R. E. Wheeler, "Epidemiology and the Control of Syphilis," *Milbank Memorial Quarterly*, 15, no. 1 (January 1937): 90–94; Theodore Rosenthal and Joseph Weinstein, "Epidemiology of Syphilis in New York City," *AJPH*, 29, no. 9 (September 1939): 1034–43.

98. Paul B. Cornely, "Health Assets and Liabilities of the Negro," *Opportunity*, 23, no. 4 (October–December 1945): 198.

99. Department of Health, Education and Welfare, "Final Report of the Tuskegee Syphilis Study Ad Hoc Panel to the Department of Health, Education and Welfare," (1973), in *Law, Science and Medicine*, edited by J. Areen et al. (Mineola, New York: Foundation Press,), 947–50; quotation is from p. 948. The best account of this tragedy remains James H. Jones, *Bad Blood: The Tuskegee Syphilis Experiment* (New York: Free Press, 1981). In the Tuskegee study a black community nurse (E. Rivers) and other black professionals perverted their intermediary, "superstructural" public health roles. On sociological processes that fed this complicity, see Martha Solomon, "The Rhetoric of Dehumanization: An Analysis of Medical Reports of the Tuskegee Syphilis Project," *The Western Journal of Speech Communication*, 49, no. 4 (Fall 1985): 233–47.

100. J. A. McFalls, Jr., "Black Fertility and VD in the U.S. Black Population, 1880–1950," *Social Biology*, 20, no. 1 (1973): 4–6; H. H. Hazen, "A Leading Cause of Death Among Negroes: Syphilis," *JNE*, 6, no. 3 (July 1937): 310–12; "Statement of Dr. Herman M. Baker, President, Indiana State Medical Association," *Investigation and Control of Venereal Diseases, Hearings, Subcommittee on Commerce, United States Senate, Seventy-Fifth Congress, Third Session on S. 3290, February 14 and 15, 1938* (Washington, D.C.: GPO, 1938) [hereafter abbreviated *Investigation and Control of VD Hearings*], 97; William J. Brown et al., *Syphilis and Other Venereal Diseases* (Cambridge: Harvard University Press, 1970), 29; Brandt, *No Magic Bullet*, 152, 154, 249, n. 83. For current perspectives on the problem of false posi-

tives caused by a variety of diseases other than syphilis—for example, narcotic addiction, systemic lupus erythematosus, as well as older age—see Beeson, *Cecil Textbook of Medicine*, 514–15; Willard Cates, Jr. and K. K. Holmes, "Sexually Transmitted Diseases," in *Maxcy-Rosenau—Public Health and Preventive Medicine*, ed. John M. Last (Norwalk, Conn.: Appleton-Century-Crofts, 1986), 271–73.

101. Lewis, *The Biology of the Negro*, 156–57.

102. Ibid., 158.

103. McFalls, Jr., "Black Fertility and VD," 6.

104. S. W. Wynne to Aaron MacGhee, 21 November 1933, rpt. in *Past, Present and Future of the Manhattan Medical Society*, 22. Dr. MacGhee was the chairman of the Manhattan Medical Society. Apparently the city arranged for the transfer of the overflow syphilis-treatment patients to the Harlem Health Center (ibid.).

105. James Summerville, *Educating Black Doctors: A History of Meharry Medical College* (University, Ala.: The University of Alabama Press, 1983), 74; Isidore Cohn, *Flint-Goodridge—An Educational Asset, Address Delivered Nov. 8, 1940 at Atlanta University, Atlanta, Ga.*, [pamphlet], *Selected Papers [of] Isidore Cohn, Vol. 2, 1930–1945, Medical Department, Tulane University*, [unpublished compendium], TUML, 6–7, 8.

106. "Statement of Dr. G. W. Bowles, York, Pa." *Investigation and Control of VD Hearings*, 92; "Statement of Dr. D. W. Byrd, Norfolk, Va.," ibid., 93.

107. "Statement of Dr. G. W. Bowles," 92; Parran, *Shadow on the Land*, 178

108. Commission On the Eradication of Syphilis of the National Medical Association, "Implications From the Viewpoint of the Negro Physician," in *Syphilis in the Negro: A Handbook for the General Practitioner, Supplement no. 15 to Venereal Disease Information*, H. H. Hazen (Washington, D.C.: GPO for U.S. Public Health Service/Federal Security Agency, 1942), Addendum, 80–81.

109. Brandt, *No Magic Bullet*, 143–47; Edward H. Beardsley, *A History of Neglect: Health Care for Blacks and Mill Workers in the Twentieth Century South* (Knoxville: University of Tennessee Press, 1987), 163–65, 171–73.

110. National Negro Health Movement with the United States Public Health Service National Negro Health Work, *WPA and Negro Health*, (n.p., 4–11 April 1937), pamphlet no. 11322, NYAM.

111. Commission on Chronic Illness, *Chronic Illness in the United States, Volume IV, Chronic Illness in a Large City—The Baltimore Study* (Cam-

bridge: The Commonwealth Fund/Harvard University Press, 1957), 12.

112. *WPA and Negro Health*, 4–5.

113. Ibid., 4.

114. Beeson et al., *Cecil Textbook of Medicine*, 566–67.

115. *WPA and Negro Health*, 8–9.

116. *Cecil Textbook of Medicine*, 318–19.

117. E. C. Tandy, "The Health Situation of Negro Mothers and Babies in the U.S.," (Washington, D.C.: U.S. Department of Labor, Children's Bureau, 1 July 1940), [rpt., 9 pp.], NYAM; E. C. Tandy, "Infant and Maternal Mortality Among Negroes," *JNE*, 6, no. 3 (July 1937): 322–49.

118. Katherine F. Lenroot, "The Health Education Program of the Children's Bureau, with Particular Reference to Negroes," *JNE*, 6, no. 3 (July 1937): 510–11.

119. Myrdal, *An American Dilemma*, 1273, n.35.

120. Ibid., 74.

121. National Negro Congress, *Official Proceedings, February 14, 15, 16, 1936* (Chicago: NNC, 1936), 5; *October 15, 16, 17, 1937* (Washington, D.C.: NNC, 1937?), Appendix: Resolutions On Health, 82–83 (includes quotation); *1938/1939* (n.p., [1939]), 4, 5. The NNC disbanded in 1940 under allegations it had become communist-infiltrated.

122. Mabel K. Staupers, *No Time For Prejudice: A Story of the Integration of Negroes in Nursing in the United States* (New York: Macmillan, 1961), 30–31, 189–90.

123. President F. D. Roosevelt to Mary McLeod Bethune, 14 January 1939; and M. M. Bethune to F. D. Roosevelt, 1 May 1939; in *The Second National Conference on the Problems of the Negro and Negro Youth, Proceedings* (n.p., 12–14 January 1939), 2–3.

124. "Report of the Evaluation Committee on Health and Housing," Dr. M. O. Bousfield, chairman (January 1939), [mimeographed, 5 pp.], L. T. Wright Papers–FCLM, 1–2.

125. Ibid., 1–2; Frances Harriet Williams to Ruth Roberts, 24 January 1939, L. T. Wright Papers–FCML. Williams was an Advisory Council member and on the staff of the National Board of the YWCA. "No progress" was reported on three recommendations: internships and residencies (3, except for a few opened at Freedmen's Hospital), a new veterans' hospital with an interracial professional staff (8), and more black personnel in the Children's Bureau's programs for handicapped children (9).

126. A. Stone to L. T. Wright, 1 November 1938; 23 January 1939; L. T. Wright, [Review of *The Negro's Struggle for Survival*, [typewritten, 1 p.], emphasis mine; L. T. Wright, [Review of *The Negro's Struggle for Survival*—second draft], [typewritten, 2 pp.]; all items in Box 1, L. T. Wright Papers–FCLM. To further demonstrate Holmes' misuse of medical data, Wright cited this example: "In spite of the large amount of work done recently on lymphogranuloma venereum, he [Holmes] quotes a study by Matas in 1896, which discusses syphilis and tuberculosis as the usual cause of rectal stricture. Rectal stricture [can be] caused by . . . lymphogranuloma venereum. Acquaintance with recent work in the field of medicine and epidemiology is almost entirely lacking. Many of his references seem to belong to ancient civilization." (L. T. Wright, [Review of *The Negro's Struggle for Survival*, first draft, 1]).

Chapter 5

1. [New York Tuberculosis And Health Association], "Statistical Survey Completed for 1939 Shows Mortality Rise in Urban Centers," *New York Tuberculosis and Health Assocation Journal*, 4, no. 3 (December 1940), 3; Atlanta Urban League, *Report on Hospital Care*, 1948 (Atlanta: The League, [c. 1949]), 23.

2. J. Yerushalmy, "The Increase in Tuberculosis Proportionate Mortality Among Nonwhite Young Adults," *PHR*, 61, no. 8 (22 February 1946): 251–58. Figures are for blacks who comprised more than 99 percent of the nation's nonwhites. Percentage of deaths caused by TB (all forms) are of all causes except pneumonia, influenza, and puerperal causes.

3. L. I. Dublin, "The Mortality from Tuberculosis Among the Race Stocks in the Southwest," Address Delivered before the Annual Meeting of the National Tuberculosis Assocation, 5 May 1941, San Antonio, Texas, Louis I. Dublin Papers–NLM, 1–2.

4. Ibid., 5. For a later example of the reservoir notion, see Leona Baumgartner, "Urban Reservoirs of Tuberculosis," *ART*, 79, no. 5 (1959): 687–89.

5. William J. Brown et al, *Syphilis and Other Venereal Diseases* (Cambridge: Harvard University Press, 1970), 112–13.

6. G. A. Spencer and R. F. Gordon, "Community Aspects of Venereal-Disease Control in Harlem," *New York State Journal of Medicine*, 46, no. 6 (March 1946): 611; Louis Lautier, "Sidelights on the Negro and the Army," *Opportunity*, 22, no. 1 (January–March, 1944): 7.

7. *Statistical Report of the the Medical Findings for the First, Second,*

Third, Fourth, Fifth, and Sixth Induction Periods in the New York City Area (Up to and Including March 15, 1941), Medical Statistics Section, Medical Division, New York City Selective Service Administration [mimeographed, 15 pp.], Series III, Box 101. C.-E. A. Winslow Papers–SLYU.

8. Atlanta Urban League, *Report on Hospital Care*, 16.

9. Spencer and Gordon, "Community Aspects of Venereal-Disease Control," 11.

10. W. A. Beck, *"Tuberculosis and the Negro," [Address for Program] Wings Over Jordan, Station WCHS, Charleston, West Virginia, July 12, 1942* [pamphlet], Box 130-10, Folder 25, Louis T. Wright Papers–MSRC, [4].

11. G. D. Cannon, "City-Wide Harlem Week [Radio Address], Station WLIB," [typewritten, 6 pp.], Box 130-11, Folder 14, Louis T. Wright Papers–MSRC, 1–3, quotation is from p. 2.

12. Ibid., 3.

13. P. B. Cornely, "Race Relations in Community Health Organization," *AJPH*, 46, no. 9 (September 1946): 984–92. This study did not identify the cities surveyed by name.

14. [American Social Hygiene Association], "Abstract of Proceedings of Conference with Negro Leaders on Wartime Problems in Venereal Disease Control, November 22, 23, 1943," [typewritten, 11 pp.], Box 70, Folder 12, Charles S. Johnson Papers–ACTU. This document is headed "Confidential," probably to keep members invited to the conference from inadvertently arousing undue alarm and public stigma concerning venereal disease among black military personnel.

15. T. K. Lawless, "Report of the Committee on Medical Facts," excerpt in "Conference with Negro Leaders on Wartime Problems," 3–4.

16. Ibid., 3.

17. "Conference with Negro Leaders on Wartime Problems," 4.

18. Ibid., 5–6; quotation is from p. 6.

19. American Social Hygiene Association, "The Development of V. D. Programs Involving the Participation of Negroes," New York City, (1945), [typewritten, 11 pp.], C. S. Johnson Papers–ACTU, 2.

20. Ibid., passim.

21. Herbert R. Edwards to C.-E. A. Winslow, 19 November 1952 [also attached typescript, 3 pp., describing the Harlem activities], C.-E. A. Winslow Papers–SLYU. Edwards was the executive director of the New York Tuberculosis and Health Association, and Winslow the prominent public

health professor and policy maker. (Mary Dempsey to Louis I. Dublin, "Tuberculosis Control Program in St. Louis City and County," 4 December 1946 [memo, 2 pp.], L. I. Dublin Papers–NLM; National Tuberculosis Association, *What Goes On in Negro Programs—A News Service Published from Time to Time by the Committee on Negro Programs of the National Tuberculosis Association*, 1, no. 10 [November 1948], [newsletter], C. S. Johnson Papers–ACTU).

22. For example, prior to 1952 most federal funds for venereal disease control were allocated to states. This meant that such factors as population density, unusual local flare-ups of the disease, and quality of service providers were usually overlooked. (Communicable Disease Center, Bureau of State Service, U.S. Department of Health, Education, and Welfare / Public Health Service, *Proceedings of the Communicable Disease Center Biennial Staff Conference, March 25–29, 1957*, CDC Library, Atlanta, Georgia, pp. B-3 to B-4.)

23. Barkev S. Sanders, "Local Health Departments—Growth or Illusion," *PHR*, 74, no. 1 (January 1959): 13–20.

24. Cornely, "Race Relations in Community Health Organization," 987.

25. P. B. Cornely, "Segregation and Discrimination in Medical Care in the United States," *AJPH*, 46, no. 9 (September 1956): 1075–81.

26. P. R. Coggs, "Race Relations Advisers—Quislings or Messiahs," *Opportunity*, 21, no. 3 (July 1943): 112. On the broader problem that post–World War II black political and professional leaders faced in brokering among the black underclass and national politics, culture, and economics, see the now-classic polemic by Harold Cruse, *The Crisis of the Negro Intellectual* (New York: Morrow, 1967).

27. I. B. Taeuber, "Change and Tansition in the Black Population of the United States," *Population Index*, 34 (April–June 1968): 121–51, cited in Daniel O. Price, "Urbanization of the Blacks," *Milbank Memorial Fund Quarterly*, 48, no. 2, Part 2 (April 1970), 52.

28. Price, "Urbanization of the Blacks," 54; A. C. Hill and F. S. Jaffe, "Negro Fertility and Family Size Preferences: Implications for Programming of Health and Social Services," in *The Negro American*, edited by Talcott Parsons and Kenneth B. Clark (Boston: Beacon Press, 1966), 206–07, 209; E. Franklin Frazier, *The Negro In the United States* (1949; New York: Macmillan, 1957), 194.

29. J. S. Collings and D. M. Clark, "General Practice Today and Tomorrow," *NEJM*, 248 (22 and 29 January 1953), in *Readings in Medical Care*, Committee on Medical Care Teaching of the Association of Teachers of Preventive Medicine (Chapel Hill: University of North Carolina Press, 1958), 214–15.

30. A. J. Harmon, "The Trend and Probable Future of Cities in Relation to Health," *AJPH*, 54, no. 5 (May 1964): 699–703; Herbert J. Gans, "The Failure of Urban Renewal," in *American Urban History*, edited by Alexander B. Callow, Jr. (New York: Oxford University Press, 1969), 570–71.

31. "A Progressive Step," *Bulletin of the Hospital Council of Greater New York*, 8, no. 5 (May 1952): 2. On discrimination in voluntary hospitals throughout other major cities during the late 1940s and 1950s, see D. C. Reitzes, *Negroes and Medicine* (Cambridge: Commonwealth Fund/Harvard University Press, 1958); and St. Claire Drake, "The Social and Economic Status of the Negro in the United States," in *The Negro American*, edited by Parsons and Clark, 26.

32. Reitzes, *Negroes and Medicine*, 333–35; H. F. Dowling, *City Hospitals: The Undercare of the Underprivileged* (Cambridge: Harvard University Press, 1982), 160–61.

33. St. Clair Drake and Horace C. Cayton, *Black Metropolis: A Study of Negro Life in a Northern City—Volume I and Volume II* (1945; New York: Harper Torchbooks, 1962, enlarged and revised ed.), Vol. 1, xlii, and Vol. 2, xix (includes quotation). While medical care needs of this inner-city went largely unmet, black cultural institutions managed to remain intact, providing sorely needed folk health practices and psychological support systems in the absence of formal hospital and psychiatric care. Cayton and Drake cited the churches of working-class blacks as an example of the cultural readjustment that blacks made to neighborhood fragmentation. "Store-front churches flourish, but [ministers] find it increasingly difficult to rent stores, since run-down business streets are being eliminated by slum clearance, and low-cost housing projects make no provision for such spiritual entrepreneurs." The larger, autonomously housed black churches simply picked up the slack by opening their services to larger and larger worship visits from this temporarily "rootless" church body. (Ibid., Vol. 2, pp. xix–xx.)

34. Louis I. Dublin, "The Problems of Negro Health as Revealed by Vital Statistics," *JNE*, 18, no. 3 (Summer 1949): 212–13; quotation is from p. 212. See also Brown et al., *Syphilis and Other Venereal Diseases*, 112–13.

35. "Statement of Dr. E. I. Robinson, President, National Medical Association, Accompanied by Dr. Paul B. Cornely," *Hearings, Committee on Education and Labor, U.S. Senate On S. 1606—Part 2, April, . . . 1946* (Washington, D.C.: GPO, 1946), 788.

36. Rayford W. Logan, "The Negro Wants First-Class Citizenship," in *What the Negro Wants*, edited by R. W. Logan (Chapel Hill: University of North Carolina Press, 1944), 15. For the impact of World War II democratic idealism on national health policy and medical education, see Cornely, "Segregation and Discrimination in Medical Care in the United States.

37. M. M. Bethune, "'Certain Inalienable Rights,'" in *What the Negro Wants*, edited by R. W. Logan, 255.

38. J. G. Scadding, "Tuberculosis as a Model for the Development of Ideas About Disease," *Society for the History of Medicine Bulletin*, 20 (1974): 4–5; quotation is from p. 5.

39. Daniel M. Fox called this faith in maximization of laboratory cures "hierarchical regionalism." See his incisive, *Health Policies, Health Politics: The British and American Experience, 1911–1965* (Princeton, N.J.: Princeton University Press, 1986).

40. P. B. Cornely, "Health Assets and Liabilities of the Negro," *Opportunity*, 23, no. 4 (October–December 1945): 198.

41. W. Montague Cobb, "The Negro and Medical Care," *Medical Care: The Twentieth Annual Debate Handbook: Volume I* (n.p., 1946), rpt., Box 130-12, Folder 11, L. T. Wright Papers–MSRC, 153.

42. Ibid., 153–54.

43. Ibid., 154–55.

44. Ernest W. Saward, "Institutional Organization, Incentives, and Change," in *Doing Better and Feeling Worse: Health in the United States*, edited by J. H. Knowles (New York: Norton, 1977), 195; V. L. Bullough and B. Bullough, *Health Care for the Other Americans* (New York: Appleton-Century-Crofts, 1982), 215. The Wagner-Murray-Dingell bill was introduced in 1943.

45. "Statement of W. Montague Cobb," *Hearings . . . On S. 1606—Part 1, April, . . . 1946*, 506, includes quote; G. D. Cannon, "Racial Contributions to American Culture—The Contributions of the Negro to Medicine," lecture at New York University, 20 December 1945, [typewritten, 28 pp.], L. T. Wright Papers–MSRC, 25; W. Montague Cobb, "The National Health Program of the NAACP," *JNMA*, 45, no. 5 (September 1953): 336.

46. Ruth Ellington James Interview with Peter M. Murray, WLIB Radio (New York), 2 May 1952, [transcript, mimeographed, 4 pp.], Peter M. Murray Papers–MSRC, 2–3; R. N. Cunningham, "Discrimination and the Doctor," *Medical Economics*, 29 (January 1952), in *Readings in Medical Care*, 180.

47. "Statement of W. Montague Cobb," 506, 507.

48. "Statement of Dr. E. I. Robinson," 787, 788, 789.

49. R. H. Shryock, *The Development of Modern Medicine* (Madison: University of Wisconsin Press, 1979), 428–30.

50. M. O. Bousfield, "Hospitals and Health Centers," paper read at

51st Session, National Medical Association, 21 August 1946, Lousiville, Kentucky, Box 130-10, Folder 43, L. T. Wright Papers–MSRC, 8–9.

51. National Medical Fellowships, Inc., *Opportunities for Negroes in Medicine* (Chicago: 1958), Box 76-10, Folder 206, P. M. Murray Papers–MSRC, 15–16. By 1958, NMF had provided grants to 246 individuals who were one-fourth of the nation's total supply of black medical specialists.

52. J. P. Guzman, ed., *Negro Year Book: A Review of Events Affecting Negro Life* (New York: William H. Wise, 1952), 168–69; Mabel K. Staupers, *No Time For Prejudice: A Story of the Integration of Negroes in Nursing in the United States* (New York: Macmillan, 1961).

53. Ronald L. Numbers described the AMA's approach to national health insurance proposals following Truman's election in 1948 as "all-out war." The expensive lobbying of the AMA was so effective during the next one and one-half decades that limited health insurance came only in 1965 when Congress passed Medicare and Medicaid. (R. L. Numbers, "The Third Party: Health Insurance in America," in *Sickness and Health in America: Readings in the History of Medicine and Public Health*, edited by R. L. Numbers and J. W. Leavitt [Madison: University of Wisconsin Press, 1978], 146–47.)

54. Charles S. Johnson, "Health," address, n.p., 1954, [typewritten, 12 pp.], Box 163, Folder 10, C. S. Johnson Papers–ACTU, 2.

55. Ibid., 8–11; quotation is from p. 11.

56. President's Commission on the Health Needs of the Nation, *Building America's Health* (Washington, D.C.: GPO, 1953), in *Readings in Medical Care*, 228–29.

57. C. S. Johnson, "Conserving the Physical Health of the Family through National Health Programs," address delivered at the Tennessee Conference on Social Work, 18 March 1954, Box 159, Folder 17, C. S. Johnson Papers–ACTU, 5.

58. Ibid., 5–8; quotation is from p. 8.

59. Detroit Commission on Community Relations, *Medical and Hospital Study Committee Report* (Detroit: The Commission, [1956]), Box 5, Leonidas H. Berry Papers–NLM, [i], 2, 3.

60. Ibid., 1, 20–21.

61. Ibid., 23.

62. Ibid., 24.

63. Drake, "The Social and Economic Status of the Negro," 27–30;

David McBride, *Integrating the City of Medicine: Blacks in Philadelphia Health Care, 1910–1965* (Philadelphia: Temple University Press, 1989), 169–74. The Chicago Commission on Human Relations did a study titled "Negro Births in Chicago's Religious Hospitals and Maternity Services—1955" which revealed systematic practices of denying services to this city's blacks. Reitzes, *Negroes and Medicine*, 108.

64. See, for example, Drake, "The Social and Economic Status of the Negro;" and Ralph Ellison, *Shadow and Act* (New York: Random House 1964), and, of course, his classic, *The Invisible Man* (New York: Random House, 1952).

65. A study in 1965 on syphilis in America society by a health policy analyst and epidemiologist illustrated the continuing tendency to overemphasize an indistinct color factor even when "Negro" was retained. Addressing why the syphilis rate of blacks appeared to be almost twenty times higher than that of whites, this researcher wrote: "In attempting to localize the main target areas of the syphilis problem, note first that the incidence of syphilis among the Negro race is extremely high compared with the white. This has always been so, both in the armed forces and in civilian society. . . . Presumably it is associated with the usual melancholy syndrome of poverty, low education, crowding, and so forth. . . . There may also be a racial reason for the higher rate among Negroes in that they have not been exposed to syphilis for as long as those of European descent who have had time to develop some immunity." (O. W. Anderson, *Syphilis and Society: Problems of Control in the United States, 1912–1964* [Chicago: Health Information Foundation, 1965], 47).

66. Rashi Fein, "An Economic and Social Profile of the Negro American," in *The Negro American*, edited by T. Parsons and K. B. Clark, 110; T. F. Pettigrew, *A Profile of the Negro American* (Princeton, N.J.: Van Nostrand, 1964), 84. As for syphilis, public health figures for 1960–61 placed the incidence of syphilis among blacks at ten times the rate of whites, and black mortality from this disease four times higher than that of whites. (Pettigrew, *A Profile of the Negro American*, 86–87).

67. P. Q. Edwards, "Is Tuberculosis Still a Problem?" *PHR*, 88, no. 6 (June–July 1973): 483–85.

68. Robert J. Anderson et al., "The Nonhospitalized Tuberculosis Patient," *PHR*, 71, no. 9 (September 1956): 888.

69. Harry F. Dowling, *Fighting Infection: Conquests of the Twentieth Century* (Cambridge: Harvard University Press, 1978), 170.

70. Shryock, *The Development of Modern Medicine*, 452–53; Monroe Lerner and O. W. Anderson, *Health Progress in the United States, 1900–1960* (Chicago: University of Chicago Press, 1963), 178–79, 183–86.

71. Anderson et al., "The Nonhospitalized Tuberculosis Patient," 888; E. T. Blomquist, "The Nonhospitalized Tuberculosis Patient," *AJPH*, 46, no. 2 (February 1956): 149.

72. Robert Glass, "Forcible Detention of Patients with Active Tuberculosis," *PHR*, 74, no. 5 (May 1959): 399–402; Edward Kupka and D. L. Gibson, "Followup of Tuberculous Recalcitrants," *PHR*, 75, no. 1 (January 1960): 21–25.

73. "Status of Tuberculosis Conference Report," *PHR*, 73, no. 11 (November 1958): 1015–20. Specific factors cited by Long as examples were hormones of the thyroid and adrenal glands; "physiological differences in the body's production" that may occur following some form of stress; mental attitudes such as "anxiety, complacency, willpower, determination, cooperativeness, hostility, care, and carelessness"; "biochemistry"; nutrition; and other diseases. (Ibid., 1016–17). There was no mention of specific TB problems of black community residents in the 1956 NTA conference summary. ("Tuberculosis [Conference]: Hospital or Home Care," *PHR*, 71, no. 9 [September 1956], 887–96).

74. Pettigrew, *A Profile of the Negro American*, 83.

75. H. M. Morais, *The History of the Negro in Medicine* (New York: Publishers Company/Association for the Study of Negro Life and History, 1968), 143–44, 159, 173–74, 182, 183; Edward H. Beardsley, *A History of Neglect: Health Care for Blacks and Mill Workers in the Twentieth Century South* (Knoxville: University of Tennessee Press, 1987), 262–64.

76. Morais, *The History of the Negro in Medicine*, 144; Beardsley, *A History of Neglect*, 262–63; McBride, *Integrating the City of Medicine*, 190.

77. W. T. Armstrong, "Address of the Speaker of the House of Delegates," Box 4, Folder 70, Joseph L. Johnson Papers–MSRC, 35.

78. *Minutes of the NMA*, 1963, Resolution #12, Box 4, Folder 71, J. L. Johnson Papers–MSRC, 25.

79. Ibid., 32; "The National Medical Association Speaks Out for Medicare, The Testimony of Dr. W. Montague Cobb, President of the NMA, before the Committee on Finance of the United States Senate," in Morais, *The History of the Negro in Medicine*, Appendix P, 266.

80. Leslie A. Falk, "The Negro American's Health and the Medical Committee for Human Rights," in *National Health Care*, edited by Ray H. Elling (Chicago: Aldine/Atherton, 1971), 79–81; James Summerville, *Educating Black Doctors: A History of Meharry Medical College* (University, Ala.: University of Alabama Press, 1983), 162.

81. A. O. Wells, Public Letter, 22 March 1965, L. H. Berry Papers–NLM.

82. Medical Committee for Human Rights, "Position Paper—National Committee of Recruitment and Medical Presence," [typewritten, 6 pp.], L. H. Berry Papers–NLM, [2].

83. John W. Hatch and Eugenia Eng, "Community Participation and Control: Or Control of Community Participation," in *Reforming Medicine: Lessons of the Last Quarter Century*, edited by V. W. Sidel and Ruth Sidel (New York: Pantheon, 1984), 228.

84. John T. English, "Is the O.E.O. Concept—the Neighborhood Health Center—the Answer?" in *Medicine in the Ghetto*, edited by J. C. Norman (New York: Appleton-Century-Crofts, 1969), 261–62; quotation is from p. 261.

85. Hatch and Eng, "Community Participation and Control," 234.

86. Ibid., 235.

87. V. L. and B. Bullough, *Health Care for the Other Americans*; George James, "Do Hospital-Based Services and Private Enterprise Offer the Best Hope for Improved Health in the Ghetto?" in *Medicine in the Ghetto*, edited by J. C. Norman, 242, includes quote. For a detailed review of the OEO's rise and fall, see A. J. Matusow, *The Unraveling of America: A History of Liberalism in the 1960s* (New York: Harper Torchbooks, 1986), 243–71; H. J. Geiger, "Community Health Centers: Health Care as an Instrument of Social Change," in *Reforming Medicine*, edited by V. W. Sidel and R. Sidel, 11–32.

Chapter 6

1. "Update: Acquired Immunodeficiency Syndrome—United States, 1981–1988," CDC, *MMWR*, 38, no. 14 (14 April 1989): 229. Annual incidence rates for AIDS among whites were 9.6 per 100,000, followed by Asians/Pacific Islanders (5.4), and American Indians/Alaskan Natives (2.2) (ibid.). The TB case rate in 1987 was 9.3 per 100,000. About two-thirds of TB cases occur among blacks, Hispanics, Asians, and Native Americans (CDC, *A Strategic Plan for the Elimination of Tuberculosis in the United States, MMWR—Supplement*, 38, no. S-3 [21 April 1989]: 1–2).

2. CDC, *A Strategic Plan for the Elimination of Tuberculosis in the United States*, 2; "Tuberculosis and Human Immunodeficiency Virus Infection: Recommendations of the Advisory Committee for the Elimination of Tuberculosis (ACET)," *MMWR*, 38, no. 14 (14 April 1989): 237; R. M. Selik, "Distribution of AIDS Cases, by Racial/Ethnic Group and Exposure Category, United States, June 1, 1981–July 4, 1988," *MMWR*, 37, no. SS-3 (July 1988): 1–3.

3. D. R. Hopkins, "AIDS in Minority Populations in the United States,"

PHR, 102 (November–December, 1987): 677; S. R. Freidman et al., "The AIDS Epidemic Among Blacks and Hispanics," *Milbank Quarterly*, 65, su2 (1987): 460–65; United States Public Health Service, U.S. Department of Health and Human Services, *AIDS—A Public Health Challenge: Vol. 2: Managing and Financing the Problem* (October 1987), chap. 9, 11; (Hispanic women total 21 percent of the female AIDS cases. [ibid.]). M. F. Rogers and W. W. Williams, "AIDS in Blacks and Hispanics: Implications for Prevention," *Issues in Science and Technology*, 3, no. 3 (Spring 1987): 90.

4. M. E. Guinan and Ann Hardy, "Epidemiology of AIDS in Women in the United States," *JAMA*, 257, no. 15 (17 April 1987): 2039–42.

5. *AIDS—A Public Health Challenge*, chap. 9, 11; Hopkins, "AIDS in Minority Populations," 677.

6. C. Everett Koop, "Teaching Children About AIDS," *Issues in Science and Technology*, 4, no. 1 (Fall 1987): 68.

7. CDC, *AIDS and Human Immunodeficiency Virus Infection in the United States: 1988 Update, MMWR—Supplement*, 38, no. S-4 (12 May 1989): 9; "Update: Acquired Immunodeficiency Syndrome—United States, 1981–1988," 235; D. S. Weinberg and H. W. Murray, "Coping with AIDS— The Special Problems of New York City," *NEJM*, 317, no. 23 (3 December 1987): 1469.

8. Freidman et al., "The AIDS Epidemic among Blacks and Hispanics," 472–73.

9. Weinberg and Murray, "Coping with AIDS," 1469.

10. G. D. Kleen et al., "Unrecognized Human Immunodeficiency Infection in Emergency Department Patients," *NEJM*, 318, no. 25 (23 June 1988): 1647.

11. "AIDS Study: A Warning of Epidemic in the Bronx," *New York Times*, 15 February 1989. This study uncovered AIDS in many of the hospital's units: obstetrics, pediatrics, methadone clinic for heroin addicts, psychiatry, dentistry, and referrals located at a neighboring shelter for the homeless.

12. O. L. Hendrix, "New York City Health and Hospitals Corporation," in *AIDS Public Policy Dimensions—Based on the Proceedings of the Conference Held January 16 and 17, 1986*, edited by John Griggs (New York: United Hospitals Fund, 1987), 140–42.

13. Lena Williams, "Inner City Under Siege: Newark Struggling to Combat AIDS," *New York Times*, 6 February 1989.

14. Alexander Moore and R. D. LeBaron, "The Case for a Haitian Origin of the AIDS Epidemic," in *The Social Dimensions of AIDS: Methods*

and Theory, edited by D. A. Feldman and T. M. Johnson (New York: Praeger, 1986), chapter 4; D. A. Feldman, "Anthropology, AIDS, and Africa," *Medical Antropology Quarterly*, 17, no. 2 (February 1986): 38–40; R. C. Gallo, forward to *A Strange Virus of Unknown Origin*, by Jacques Leibowitch (New York: Ballantine Books, 1985), xi–xii; F. J. Bennett, "AIDS As A Social Phenomenon," *Social Science and Medicine*, 25, no. 6 (1987): 529–30. For an example in European literature, see Leibowitch, *A Strange Virus of Unknown Origin*.

15. For a balanced introduction to the serious methodological errors inherent in epidemiologic and behavioral health research that use unqualified race terms, see L. O. Watkins, "Epidemiology of Coronary Health Disease in Black Poplulations: Methodologic Proposals," *American Heart Journal*, 108, no. 3, part 2 (September 1984): 635–40; Richard Cooper, "Race, Disease and Health," in *Health, Race & Ethnicity*, edited by Thomas Rathwell and David Phillips (London: Croom Helm, 1986), 21–79; D. Y. Wilkinson and Gary King, "Conceptual and Methodological Issues in the Use of Race as a Variable: Policy Implications," *Milbank Quarterly*, 65, supp. 1 (1987): 56–71.

16. For examples of the views of African and Haitian officials and health care field-workers, see "Prepared Statement of Ambassador Wanume Kibedi, Permanent Representative of Uganda to the United Nations," United States House, 89th Congress, Select Committee on Hunger, *AIDS and the Third World: The Impact on Development—Hearings, Washington, D.C., June 30, 1988*, Microfiche Serial no. 100-29, 63–64; "Prepared Statement of Michael S. Gerber, Ph.D., President, African Medical & Research Foundation, AMREF/USA," ibid., 104–05; and Ary Bordes, *Un Médecin Raconte* (Port-au-Prince, Haiti: Editions Henri Deschamps, 1989), 295–98. For a critique of the postulation that AIDS "began" in Africa, see P. Katner and G. A. Pankey, "Evidence for a Euro-American Origin of Human Immunodeficiency Virus (HIV)," *JNMA*, 79, no. 10 (1987): 1068–72. For studies criticizing as faulty the early epidemiological data suggesting endemic and pandemic AIDS in Africa, see *AIDS in Africa; The Social and Policy Impact*, edited by Norman Miller and R. C. Rockwell (Lewiston, N.Y./Queenston, Ont.: Edwin Mellen Press, 1988); and R. C. and R. J. Chirimuuta, *AIDS, Africa and Racism* (Stanhope Nr. Burton-on-Trent, U.K.: Bretby House, 1987). As for the medical anthropological weaknesses of the African/Haitian-origins-of-AIDS argument, see John Kreniske, review of *The Social Dimensions of AIDS*, by D. A. Feldman and T. M. Johnson, in *Medical Anthropology Quarterly*, New Series, 3, no. 1 (March 1989): 84.

17. *AIDS—A Public Health Challenge*, chap. 9, 16; Hopkins, "AIDS in Minority Populations," 680–81.

18. Office of Science and Technology Policy, Executive Office of the President, *A National Effort to Model AIDS Epidemiology—Report of a Workshop Held at Leesburg, Virginia, July 25–29, 1988*, 36–37.

19. Rogers and Williams, "AIDS in Blacks and Hispanics," 93; Richard Goldstein, "The Hidden Epidemic: AIDS and Race," *Village Voice*, 10 March 1987.

20. Michael Gorman and David Mallon, "The Role of a Community-Based Health Education Program in the Prevention of AIDS," *Medical Anthropology*, 10, nos. 2–3 (1989): 159–60.

21. Eric Sandstrom, "Community Efforts to Combat HIV in Sweden," *AIDS in Children, Adolescents & Hetereosexual Adults: An Interdisciplinary Approach to Prevention*, edited by R. F. Schinazi and A. J. Nahmias (New York: Elsevier, 1988) 91–93.

22. Ibid. STDs are sexually-transmitted diseases.

23. *AIDS—A Public Health Challenge*, chap. 9, 16–17.

24. Ibid.; New York State Assembly, *Committee On Health, Annual Report—1987*, 11; "New York City AIDS Hospital Strives to Become Model for the Nation," *American Hospital Association News*, 25 May 1987.

25. Government of the District of Columbia, Mayor's Interagency Task Force on Acquired Immune Deficiency Syndrome, *AIDS: Fiscal Years 1987 and 1988—District of Columbia Comprehensive City-Wide Response Plan* (n.p.: [1988]), 7–11.

26. Williams, "Inner City Under Siege."

27. S. C. Joseph, "Community-Based Resources in New York City," in *AIDS in Children*, edited by Schinazi and Nahmias, 88–90.

28. "Black Clergy to Preach About AIDS," *New York Times*, 10 June 1989. A review of other black community-based activities in New York City aimed at reducing the AIDS threat is provided in Ernest Quimy and S. R. Friedman's, "Dynamics of Black Mobilization against AIDS in New York City," *Social Problems*, 36, no. 4 (October 1989): 403–15.

29. "The Black Coalition On AIDS," [informational handout (2 pp.) at "AIDS: Health Department Leadership and Community Response—National Conference," San Francisco Department of Public Health, 4–7 November 1987]; quote is from p. 2. "San Francisco Blacks At High Risk For AIDS, Study Shows," *San Francisco Sun Reporter*, 29 July 1987.

30. On negative views in the black community toward homosexuality, see Thad Martin, "AIDS: Is It a Major Threat to Blacks," *Ebony*, 40 (October 1985): 92; Lynn Norment, "The Truth About AIDS," *Ebony*, 42 (April 1987): 128; Laura B. Randolph, "The Hidden Fear: Black Women, Bisexuals and the AIDS Risk," *Ebony*, 43 (January 1988): 123; F. R. Lee, "Black Doctors Urge Study of Factors in Risk of AIDS," *New York Times*, 21 July 1989.

31. *AIDS—A Public Health Challenge*, chap. 7, 35, includes quote; Mervyn Silverman, "Community-Based Services: The San Francisco Experience," in *AIDS in Children*, edited by Schinazi and Nahmias, 83–84.

32. *AIDS—A Public Health Challenge*, chap. 7, 35; "Update: AIDS—United States, 1981–1988," 3; Gorman and Mallon, "The Role of a Community-Based Health Education Program in the Prevention of AIDS," 161.

33. Hopkins, "AIDS in Minority Populations," 680.

34. On the issue of institutionalized dominance of black women by the medical care sector, see Helen Rodriguez-Trias, "The Women's Health Movement," in *Reforming Medicine*, edited by V. W. Sidel and Ruth Sidel, (New York: Pantheon, 1984), 106–26; D. K. Newman et al., *Protest, Politics, and Prosperity* (New York: Pantheon, 1978), 187–206; Sally Guttmacher, review of *Women and AIDS* by Diane Richardson (New York: Methuen, 1988), *Medical Anthropology Quarterly*, 3, no. 1 (March 1989): 85–87 and the literature cited in *But Some of Us Are Brave: Black Women's Studies*, edited by G. T. Hull et al. (Old Westbury, N.Y.: Feminist Press, 1982), 103–114.

35. Williams, "Inner City Under Siege."

36. Joyce Wallace, "Discussion—Community Resources," *AIDS in Children*, edited by Schinazi and Nahmias, 104.

37. See, for instance, W. H. Watson, "Folk Medicine and Older Blacks in the Southern United States," *Black Folk Medicine: The Therapeutic Significance of Faith and Trust*, edited by W. H. Watson (New Brunswick, N.J.: Transaction Books, 1984), 53–66; Hans A. Baer, *The Black Spiritual Movement: A Religious Response to Racism* (Knoxville: University of Tennessee Press, 1988); A. H. Jenkins, "Black Families: The Nurturing of Agency," *Black Families in Crisis: The Middle-Class*, edited by A. F. Coner-Edwards and Jeanne Spurlock (New York: Brunner/Mazel, 1988), 115–28; and a study of maternal health services in Louisiana by M. C. Ward, *Poor Women, Powerful Men: America's Great Experiment in Family Planning* (Boulder, Colo.: Westview Press, 1986).

38. Lee, "Black Doctors Urge Study of Factors in Risk of AIDS."

39. P. M. Boffey, "U.S. Drops AIDS Study in Community Protests," *New York Times*, 17 August 1988.

40. Norment, "The Truth About AIDS," 130.

Index

acquired immune deficiency syndrome, see AIDS

African-Americans, *see* blacks

AIDS, 1, 5–6, 124, 126, 157, 159, 169–71; black community's response to, 166–71; compared to TB and syphilis epidemics, 160–63; and IV-drug use, 164, 165, 168; state programs for control of, 165; Sweden's program for control of, 164–65.

AIDS Health-Care Response Plan (District of Columbia), 166

Ainu (of Japan), 50

alcoholism, 20

Alexander, Virginia M., 44–45, 65

American Child Association, 63

American Hospital Association, 152

American Journal of Dermatology & Genito-Urinary Diseases, 18

AMA, *see* American Medical Association

American Medical Association (AMA), 18, 79, 142–43, 145, 152; *Hygeia,* 111

American Nurses' Association, 145

American Public Health Association: *The Nation's Health,* 111

antibiotics: early researchers, 20

American Review of Tuberculosis (ART), 99

American Social Hygiene Association. See ASHA

Anderson, Peyton F., 111–12

Armstrong Association (Philadelphia), 39

Armstrong, W. T., 153

ASHA (American Social Hygiene Association), 130–34

atherosclerosis, *see* heart disease(s)

Atlanta University Conference for the Study of the Negro Problems, 11, 12, 23–24

Augustine, D. L., 57–58, 100

Baggott, B. T., 95

Baltimore: city hospitals of, 44; *see also* black communities; tuberculosis-control programs and facilities

Barnett, Claude A., 98, 121

Barnhart, Kenneth, 43

Bean, Robert B., 24, 100

Beck, William A., 128–29

behavioral disorders, 3

Best, Ella, 121

Bethune, Mary McLeod, 122, 131, 139

Birmingham (Alabama), 13

Black Coalition On AIDS (San Francisco), 167

black children, 37, 57, 64, 73–75, 87–88, 120; *see also* infant and maternal health; Knox, Jr., J. H. Mason

black communities: of Baltimore, 105; biracial organization of, 76–77; and growth of inner-city populations, 135–38; and OEO programs, 155–56; voluntary health campaigns in, 10, 25–28; *see also* culture; Great Migration

black hospitals, 24–26, 27, 45, 54, 62, 65, 70, 75–76, 78–79, 93, 116, 123, 137, 142, 198n.3;